4th Edition

The English Speaker's

Guide to Medical Care in Mexico

by

Monica Rix Paxson

4th Edition

The English Speaker's Guide to Medical Care in Mexico

by Monica Rix Paxson

Copyright © 2010-2017

ISBN: 978-1-942790-04-4

Book Website: http://DoctorsAndHospitalsinMexico.com/
Author's Website: http://monicarixpaxson.com/

Published by Relentlessly Creative Books, USA Publisher's Website:
http://relentlesslycreative.com/

Publisher's Email: books@relentlesslycreative.com

Other titles by Monica Rix Paxson

The English Speaker's Guide to Doctors & Hospitals in Mexico
Talking2Trees & Other True Transdimensional Tales
Ponzi: The Prince of Pi Alley
The Fabulous Money-Making Garage Sale Kit
Dead Mars, Dying Earth
The Trouble with Level Three

Photo & Editorial Credits

We gratefully acknowledge and thank the following photographers and editorial contributors. Cover photos by Magai Gómez / MAGAPIX. Interior photos, IMSS by Javier de la Mora, Arnica By Bernd Haynold - Own work, CC BY-SA 2.5, https://commons.wikimedia.org/w/index.php?curid=208617 Editorial contributions published with permission from IAMAT, Mexico Mike, Rolly Brooks, and Paul and Linda Kurtzweil of Two Expats Living in Mexico

Permission has been obtained wherever the source can be located and has responded to our requests, however we are always happy to make corrections, include omissions or to update information. books@relentlesslycreative.com.

I'd also like to extend special thanks to Matthew Harrup, Publisher of Mexperience.com, the definitive web resource for authoritative information on Mexico, for his commitment to excellence, his editing abilities and his friendship.

Dedication

The Hospital de Jesús Nazareno in Mexico City will soon be 500 years old. As the oldest hospital in North America, the 4th edition of The English Speaker's Guide to Medical Care in Mexico is dedicated to honoring the 500th anniversary of its founding.

Disclaimer

The English Speaker's Guide to Medical Care in Mexico is not intended to give medical advice. It is a reference guide that is designed to help readers to understand the medical culture of Mexico and to find resources that provide the kind of care they are looking for.

This book provides listings and links for informational purposes only. For example, when laws are cited, the intention is to provide information about the law, not to act as a lawyer giving legal advice. Similarly, when medical information is offered here, it is not to act as a medical professional giving medical advice.

People who are using this resource are responsible for using their own judgment to determine the medical/surgical qualifications of any individual, medical service provider or medical care facility listed. You should also seek the advice of a medical professional before taking any medicine, including traditional medicinal plants.

Monica Rix Paxson has not independently reviewed or confirmed the information provided by the governmental or medical organizations that are the sources of information for this publication and does not warrant the accuracy of the information provided in this guide. In no event shall Monica Rix Paxson, Relentlessly Creative Books, her web publishers, printers or book distributors be liable for any decision made or taken by you or another based on this information.

Monica Rix Paxson has no control over emergency response, ambulance service or local emergency phone numbers. Mexico's new national 911 system may or may not work on cellular phones. Cellular phones may not be in range of cellular service in an emergency. Responders may not speak English.

Because Monica Rix Paxson is a researchers and writer and not a healthcare provider, she will not answer medical questions. Your questions about treatment in Mexico should be directed to a licensed medical professional.

Table of Contents

Welcome to the 4th Edition

When the first edition of *The English Speaker's Guide to Medical Care in Mexico* was published in 2010, the primary questions expatriates had were about the quality of care. Now the questions are more specific: Where can I find my medicine? Can I use Medicare here? The quality issue has been resolved. Care in Mexico is good to excellent. It is also affordable.

I am very proud of the amazing achievements Mexico has made in fulfilling on its promise to provide healthcare for everyone. Coming from a land where the healthcare system is hopelessly broken and people live in fear of not being able to afford care (or facing bankruptcy for having received it), I would like to acknowledge my beloved adopted country for making medical care a priority for all its citizens and for graciously and generously including those of us fortunate foreigners who are able to participate in your public health system.

It is not surprising to me that *International Living* magazine has named Mexico the best retirement destination in the world in 2017. That is, to a great extent, because they also rank Mexico in the top four countries with the best health care in the world (along with Malaysia, Costa Rica and Colombia).

Mexico made a commitment to the admirable goal of providing care for everyone and continuous quality improvement. Mexico has delivered on the promise. This is a remarkable achievement.

¡Felicidades y gracias México! México es el mejor del mundo.

Tips for Using This Book

Because *The English Speaker's Guide to Medical Care in Mexico* is available in print, Kindle and pdf ebook versions, all hyperlinks are indicated by endnote references (small numbers, like footnotes, only listed at the end of the book rather than the bottom of the page).

You will also see many cross references shown with the word "*See*" in brackets. If you are reading an interactive version of the book, a click on the cross reference may take you to that section of the book depending on the capabilities of the device you are using.

Because there is so much reference material in this book, you will find most it in a series of 17 appendices at the back of the book. Cross references indicate related appendices. They are also listed in the Table of Contents.

By separating the reference material from the narrative in this edition, I hope to make this book a more enjoyable reading experience. You can learn a lot about Mexico through the lens of its medical system and how medicine is practiced.

The two-page Table of Contents does not cover all of the topics covered in this book. You will find that the index helpful if you are looking for a specific topic. [*See Index*]

Why I Wrote This Book

For years, even before I moved to Mexico, I've belonged to an expat e-group in Cuernavaca, Morelos where I live these days. Over time I saw that medical care was one of the major topics that expats in Mexico ask each other about. Of course, most of us don't think about medical care until we need it, but when I started to research, I discovered that about 25% of all travelers have some kind of medical need during their travels. With over 1 million English-speaking expats living in Mexico and 22 million tourists visiting Mexico every year, I could see there was a need for this guide.

But in truth, my interest was also very personal and it started with my first encounter with the medical system in Mexico.

Keep in mind that I'm from Chicago where I was covered by a corporate health insurance plan, so I didn't worry about hospitalization. But the annual deductible of $2000 and co-pays for every doctor's visit were painful at times.

I got into the habit of dealing with that $2000 annual deductible mostly by avoiding medical attention altogether. Why? Because it seemed like between meeting the annual deductible and the pharmaceuticals that seemed to always be part of the package, it was seldom under $150 US to see a doctor, and frequently more. Once I paid over $1000 US to have a routine bladder infection treated.

I also never felt good about seeing a doctor. Between the waiting room, undressing in the examining room, wearing the paper gown and a sense of rush, it was typically a cold and unpleasant experience.

So, on a visit to Mexico City I was reluctant to seek medical attention when I wasn't feeling well. After a couple of days of complaining, the friend I was visiting asked me for the third time why I didn't go to the doctor. I finally confessed. I was afraid it might be expensive. He was completely puzzled by my reluctance and offered to pay.

The place we went was pretty basic: a waiting room with no receptionist and a single doctor practicing next to an associated pharmacy (a common arrangement I was to later discover) but the doctor seemed to be much warmer and more patient than I had experienced in years. She seemed to genuinely care and the treatment she outlined seemed reasonable.

All of this was reassuring, but when I left, prescription in hand, the big shock was the bill: 25 pesos, or roughly $2 US at the time. And the medications I got were both inexpensive (three of them for a total of $6 US) and effective. I was better within hours.

I was so shocked that I was moved to tears. Here I had just seen a doctor who didn't rush me, seemed to care, gave me a reasonable diagnosis and carefully explained the prescribed treatment for $2? I was accustomed to doing without even minimal care to avoid the financial burden, but here in Mexico I was receiving care for next to nothing.

My appreciation for medical care in Mexico has grown ever since and I'm glad I'll have an opportunity to share more about that with you. So, you might say that I wrote this book out of gratitude because I am grateful.

Who This Guide is For

This *Guide to Medical Care in Mexico* is written for English speakers who are traveling or living in Mexico. Thus many of the specific topics and references given are those that would be of interest to people in the United States, Canada and the United Kingdom. It is designed to help those whose knowledge of the Spanish language may be limited or non-existent and who may be new to the country and culture of Mexico. Most readers will fall into one of seven categories, each with specific interests and concerns. This guide is designed to help you if you fall into one of these categories.

You are a Traveler

You are interested in having quick, easy access to information. Perhaps you have specific health concerns and unanswered health and safety questions: Will you be able to find emergency treatment? Will it be safe to travel with a chronic condition? Will your health insurance from home cover medical treatment? What kind of vaccines or preventative measures do you need to take to be safe in Mexico?

You are a Retiree

You are planning to or have retired and are considering making your home in Mexico full time or at least part of the year as a snowbird. You want to make sure you can find adequate, affordable medical care. You need to take care of yourself and possibly family members. You need to have all of your medical needs addressed from routine checkups to major surgery. You need to carefully consider end- of-life issues such as live-in help and assisted living.

You are a Businessperson

Your work requires that you visit Mexico and you need to know how to get any emergency or routine care you may need far from home. Perhaps you are considering starting, expanding or investing in a new business in Mexico. You need to know that your family and employees will be able to access good quality treatment where you are planning to do business. You may also need to know that medical treatment, insurance and other costs will not be a barrier to doing business in Mexico.

You are Critically Ill

You are seeking alternative forms of treatment. Perhaps you have been given a terminal diagnosis or have tried all the available recommended treatments in your own country. You may be looking for places that offer experimental or alternative treatments that aren't available at home.

You Need Affordable Medical Options

Typically, you are looking for lower-cost treatment or elective surgeries. You may be seeking long-term care for a family member or fertility treatments to expand your family. Perhaps you are uninsured or underinsured and there is a standard procedure that you desperately need. Perhaps you want to have a cosmetic or other surgery that your current health insurance won't pay for and you are seeking lower- cost alternatives. You may be seeking affordable live-in care or a resident facility for an aging parent and your home country doesn't offer acceptable options at a price you can afford.

You are an Expat or Moving to Mexico

You are moving to Mexico or maybe you already live there but you don't have a doctor or need to find help. In either case, you haven't found the kind of medical care you need yet and you aren't sure what's available, how to pay for it or how to go about finding specialized treatment or affordable medical insurance options. You may have a chronic condition, a medication you take regularly or mobility issues you'll need to consider.

You are a Disabled US Veteran

Your disability has been certified by the Veteran's Administration, but you are finding that your quality of life is sub-standard in the US. You cannot afford decent housing or you are having trouble finding good affordable help. You are interested in knowing more about a little-known government program that will pay your medical costs in Mexico and might you consider life in Mexico if you could receive all the benefits you are entitled to, have full coverage for your medical expenses and improve the quality of your life. [*See Foreign Medical Program for Disabled US Veterans*]

How This Guide Will Help You

The **Guide to Medical Care in Mexico** is designed to give you the best possible experience of medical care in Mexico. Wherever you are, this guide will help you to make more informed decisions that are appropriate to your needs, your circumstances and your financial resources. It is intended to be both reassuring and realistic.

For example, without a doubt Mexico has many well-trained physicians including many specialists, many large, modern, spacious, well-equipped, sparkling-clean hospitals and high-quality, easily accessible pharmaceuticals. And, remarkably, all of this is available at comparatively low cost.

This doesn't mean that there also aren't instances of unqualified physicians, inadequate facilities, etc., in Mexico. But if you are armed with an understanding of how things work in general (and specific information whenever possible), you will better know the range of options available to you.

Finding the Care You Need

This guide focuses on how you can get the care you need but it does not contain an evaluation of individual medical practitioners. After all, Mexico is a large country with thousands of cities, *pueblos* and *colonias* and a population in the many millions. Its highly developed medical system has thousands of institutions and health care providers and information changes all the time. New doctors are trained, they move, they retire, etc.

Overall, the medical system in Mexico has approximately 20,000 primary care facilities and 4,000 hospitals. And while there many approaches to finding good care, there is no single comprehensive evaluation that takes into consideration the myriad of options available in Mexico.

If you are seeking a referral to an English speaking physician, specialist or a hospital where you are likely to find help in English, you might want to consider purchasing the companion book to this one: *The English Speaker's Guide to Doctors & Hospitals in Mexico*.[1] It lists names and contact information by location. [*See Appendix A: The English Speaker's Guide to Doctors & Hospitals in Mexico*]

So, whether you are a traveler, doing business in Mexico, considering Mexico as a place to retire or a long-time resident who has expatriated from the USA, Canada, Europe or elsewhere, you should find this guide to be a helpful companion.

Whether you are a fluent speaker of Spanish, or know nothing more than "hola" and "gracias," this publication could potentially help you communicate effectively with others even in a crisis. And because many readers are considering Mexico as a permanent full- or part-time home, you need to know that your health needs can be met at every stage of life.

The History of Medicine in Mexico

Many people are surprised to learn that both the first medical school and the first hospital in North America were founded in Mexico City. 500 years ago. Like Mexico today, early Mexicans had many hospitals. In the Western Hemisphere, modern medicine began in Mexico.

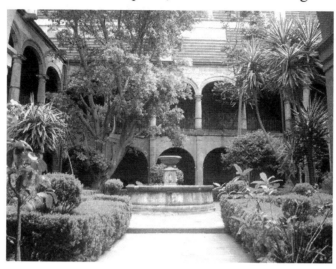

Courtyard of the 500-year-old *Hospital de Jesús Nazareno* in Mexico City

The first hospital in North America was undoubtedly built in Mexico City, and most agree that it was *Hospital de la Purísima Concepción*, later renamed *Hospital de Jesús Nazareno* and frequently call simply Hospital de Jesús, (although there are two other hospitals that were built around the same time in Mexico). It is still standing and in operation today as it has been since 1524, and nearly a century before the Pilgrims arrived on North American shores aboard the Mayflower in 1620.

The first hospital was ordered built and funded by Cortés, in gratitude (as he declared in his will) "for the graces and mercies God had bestowed on him in permitting him to discover and conquer New Spain and in expiation or satisfaction for any sins he had committed, especially those that he had forgotten, or any burden there might be on his conscience for which he could not make special atonement." ("I wonder what could possibly have been on that man's conscious?" the author asks with bitter irony.)

Mexico has always been a place of medical firsts. For example, the first medical book printed in the New World was printed in 1570 in Mexico City on presses that had just arrived in New Spain thirty years earlier. Entitled *Opera Medicinalia*, by Francisco Bravo and published by Pedro Ocharte, there is only one known copy. It is safely housed in *La Biblioteca José María Lafragua* at the *Benemérita Universidad Autónoma de Puebla* in Mexico and has been digitized by the *Primeros Libros* project where all can view it online. [2]

While I find this part of Mexico's history fascinating, it is important to remember that the history of medical practice in Mexico extends much further back than the arrival of Cortez. Not only was the practice of medicine highly evolved before the arrival of Europeans, indigenous Mexicans also published medical "books" (codices) before the invention of the printing press.

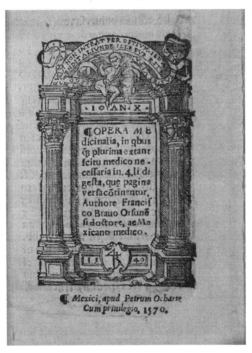

Title page for *Opera Medicinalia*

When the Spaniards arrived in 1521 there was already a flourishing tradition of healing arts including surgery, cures, herbs, minerals, baths, animals, etc. The Aztecs were far cleaner and more enlightened about health and medical practices than the Spaniards were Illustrations of many of these plants and practices appear in pre-Columbian documents (codices). In one, 272 plant varieties with curative powers are illustrated, in another, there are 142 healing herbs, and yet another provides 73 more. Perhaps even more remarkable is how many of these medicinal plants were effective and are still used in traditional indigenous medical practice today. [*See Traditional Medicine*]

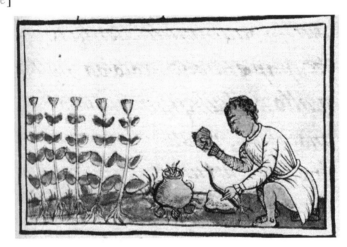

Aztec codice showing cultivation and preparation of an herbal medicine

Navigating the Modern Mexican Medical System

The International Nature of Medicine

Finding and evaluating medical practitioners in Mexico is not much different than it would be in your home country. In fact, the world of medicine is increasingly international and medical careers are highly mobile. For example, many hospitals in the USA are staffed primarily by foreign-trained doctors. Both doctors born in the US and foreign born have been trained all over the world. And many of the physicians and dentists practicing in Mexico have received at least part of their training in the USA, Canada or Europe.

Conversely, Mexico has many respected medical schools that attract students from world over. [*See Medical Training in Mexico*] Many of these students chose Mexico as a place for training both because of the quality of the education, the affordability, weather, beaches, etc. In other words, doctors train in Mexico for many of the same reasons people consider Mexico an excellent place to live. So, Mexico not only trains its own physicians, you may be surprised to discover that your physician in the US, Canada or the United Kingdom received their training, or some part of it, in Mexico.

As part of the scientific community, there are many medical professionals who speak some level of English because English is internationally recognized as the language of preference for the sciences.

You may also find that some practitioners have staff members hired particularly for their English-speaking ability, especially in those cities and regions that have large ex-patriot communities or those who cater to the medical tourist.

Expect Differences

You will find many similarities between medical treatment in your home country and treatment in Mexico, particularly in the large cities. In fact, because of global trends, many urban medical practices look and feel virtually the same as those in the USA, Canada or the United Kingdom. But for much of Mexico, you may find differences that are rather startling.

Many people consider the differences to be positive—to the point that it would be hard to be without them. Some, expecting everything to be exactly like it was in their home country, mistake the differences for bad practice. It's important to remember that you are in another culture and you are the one that is "out of place" here. Be patient and you too may soon understand why so many expats love their doctors in Mexico and find medical care there to be more humane.

If you are planning to spend any time in Mexico, it is a good idea to form a relationship with a primary care physician or *médico de cabecera*. Ideally you can get a recommendation from someone you know and trust. However, there are many approaches you can take to locate candidates and this guide suggests lots of them. But once you've made an appointment (or dropped by during office hours, which is often acceptable and there are consultancies where this is standard practice) [*See Farmacias Similares*] don't expect your visit to be exactly like those you are accustomed to.

More Hands-On Care

One of the first things you may notice when you are at a doctor's office is that physicians spend much more time talking to and examining their patients. The approach is more personal and literally hands-on. Practitioners rely more on their experience, direct contact with the body (palpation, stethoscope, etc.) and listening to what you have to say than batteries of tests, at least initially. The level of personal concern and physical intimacy may be almost shocking to those who have had a lifetime of highly impersonal, rushed, high-technology medical care.

And the level of personal care doesn't end at the office door. Many general practitioners still make house calls for their ill and housebound patients, a practice that ended in the US in the 1950s. Gone is the rush to get you out the door or out of the hospital quickly, and the sense of limited time and limited caring.

Less "Machine Medicine"

While the description that follows may vary a great deal depending on where you are being treated, you may also notice that the office and the examining room routine lack some of the things that you are used to expecting in a medical office. For example, there may not be any receptionist, reception desk or physician's assistants. You may not be asked to complete lengthy pre-examination paperwork. It may be very minimal or non-existent.

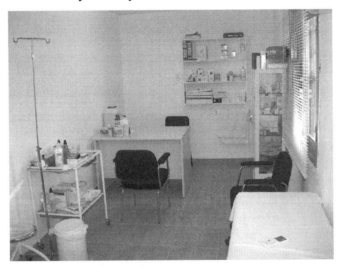

A typical *consultorio*

There may only be a single examining room, or perhaps the examining room will be a combination of consultancy, with a desk and chairs in the room where exams are done. (Of course, you may find a new clinic with multiple examining rooms as well, but don't be surprised if things aren't quite what you are accustomed to.)

You may or may not be asked to disrobe entirely and wear a gown as you typically would in the USA or Canada for even the most minor problems. It may be considered adequate to simply expose the parts that are needed—to pull out your shirttails, lift your shirt or unzip your pants. These are cultural differences, not signs of malpractice.

Nearly all tests will be done off-premises, including blood work. So, you will probably not see a technician in the doctor's office to draw blood, and if blood tests, ultrasound, X-rays, CAT scan, MRIs, mammography, etc., are required, you will be directed where to go for them, usually a nearby lab. (Even dental offices often have X-rays done in an external laboratory.) In fact, the only equipment you may see in a general practitioner's office may be very basic: stethoscope, blood-pressure cuff, flashlight, tongue depressors, cotton balls, etc.

But the differences don't end there. When you are done with the visit, the bill may be for as little as 25 pesos (about $2 for a pharmacy-owned clinic) [*See Farmacias Similares*] to a sky-high maximum of perhaps as much as $30–60 US for a private urban practice or perhaps as much as $100 US for a visit with a highly trained specialist such as a cardiologist. Overall, medical expenses will be 30% or less of what they are in the US.

Why Medical Costs Are Lower in Mexico

A 20-year-old young man recently posted his $55,000 hospital bill for an appendectomy at a hospital in Sacramento, California on Reddit with this comment: "I never truly understood how much healthcare in the US costs until I got appendicitis in October. I'm a 20-year-old guy. Thought other people should see this to get a real idea of how much an unpreventable illness costs in the US".

What followed was a firestorm of response with over 10,000 comments posted. Even with coverage through his father's insurance policy, this young man was saddled with over $11,000 in debt that will take him years to repay.

I think we can all agree that emergency procedures like appendectomies are not only essential, they must be handled quickly and near home. But why is it so expensive to have what is a routine surgical procedure in the U.S? Many would argue that it is because of the quality of the care provided. The implication is essentially "you get what you pay for." But is that true? For example, in Mexico medical care costs a fraction of what it does in the USA. Does that imply that the quality of care is lower? Exactly why is care less expensive in Mexico?

While it is a complex issue, and some of the reasons simply have to do with the overall economic differences, here are a few reasons that simply pertain to the medical culture of Mexico:

Lower Salaries

Physicians in Mexico do not typically earn six-figure salaries. According to the New York Times,[3] the average physician in Mexico earns $25,000 per year. Earnings in Mexico are lower across the entire spectrum of jobs and this is just as true for doctors and other medical professionals. For example, according to World Salaries,[4] professional nurses in Mexico earn just under $550 per month. But there's more to it than that.

No Student Debt

Most doctors in Mexico do not start their professional careers needing to pay off student debt. Bloomberg reports that the median student debt for a medical student in the USA in 2012 was $170,000 US, but for some institutions it will be much higher. This does not include the student debt from undergraduate school, nor interest. Patients in the USA, their employers and insurance companies, ultimately pay these student loans. In Mexico, many medical students study at free public universities or in private universities with much lower tuition.

No Malpractice Insurance

Unlike medical practice in the USA, for example, physicians do not typically order additional, frequently expensive and questionably unnecessary medical tests to proactively defend themselves against anticipated lawsuits. Doctors in Mexico do not purchase malpractice insurance (so there is no incentive for patients to sue for malpractice) and thus saving the $4,000-20,000 US in annual malpractice insurance that doctors in the USA typically pay.

Doctors are not driven to generate high-volume, over-booked medical practices in Mexico by the economic demands of having the latest equipment, expensive malpractice insurance and the need for additional staffing to bill insurance companies, manage complex scheduling, the flow of patients into and out of examining rooms and to provide 'witnesses' during exams with female patients.

No Third Parties

Furthermore, in Mexico a physician more typically owns his or her medical practice. There are few HMOs, PPOs or other corporate entities (and their shareholders) expecting and extracting a share of profits.

The attention of physicians in Mexico is more typically fully on the patient with fewer distractions by pharmaceutical representatives and phone calls from pharmacists in the background—and the need to hire people to manage those intrusions. And since the physician has lower expenses and all the money goes directly to the physician, you, the patient, have lower medical costs.

While the examples cited above are just part of the whole picture, it should be clear that it is entirely possible to offer world-class medical care at affordable prices because well-trained physicians are paid less and there are no complex layers of corporate interests grabbing profits. And, while you have no choice where to get help when you need an appendix removed in a hurry, in many cases you do have a choice of where to go for healthcare–and more people than ever are considering medical travel to Mexico as an option.

You Are the Keeper of the Records

Another significant difference between many medical practices in Mexico and what is typical in the US, Canada and Europe: the physician may not keep medical records. You are expected to keep your own and to bring them with you. If you are insured under Instituto Mexicano del Seguro Social (IMSS) or *Seguro Popular,* you will also need to bring your *carnet*, the little booklet or the ID you are issued with your personal information and appointment record. Mexicans typically carry their medical records in their *mica*, a plastic envelope.

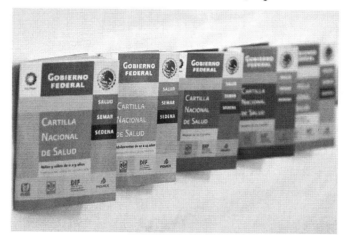

With IMSS, your *carnet* is your medical record

While you may be asked for a brief history and information about allergies to medications, unless you are in the hospital there will not typically be a chart recording your medical history, a folder, nor even a record of the prescriptions that you have been given in many general practices. Therefore, it is helpful for you to bring your own health history with you and to keep a record of any prescriptions you are given, etc.

Make it a practice to maintain your own records. If you are in the hospital, it is a good idea to keep copies of test results, x-rays, etc., even though hospitals will keep a medical record with your chart. But with public healthcare, your attending physician in the hospital and primary care physician may be different people, so you will want to be able to help any physician you are working with to get up to speed quickly.

Included in this guide is a form you may wish to complete with some standard health history information. Use it as the beginning of your own health-history file. It asks questions that will help your current physician determine if you will need any preventative vaccines. You can also ask your current physician for a photocopy or digital copy of your records to bring to Mexico. [*See Appendix B: Medical History Form*] [5]

As more records are digitized today, even X-rays, mammograms and CT scans may be available to you in digital format (ask for them in Medical Records at the hospital or facility where the scans were done) and conveniently stored on a CD, DVD or USB thumb drive. This could be vitally important in the future, particularly if you have a serious or chronic health problem.

In fact, if you have complex medical issues, and you are planning a move to Mexico, you might even consider having your history translated to Spanish simply to assure that the medical personnel you meet will be able to understand your needs quickly.

In any case, you can expect to take a new level of responsibility for maintaining and updating your medical records.

The Mexican Healthcare System

A Marriage of Public & Private Institutions

The Government of Mexico offers its citizens, by constitutional mandate, universal health care through a complex system of public and private funding. Although millions of people are covered by public insurance (55% of the population) through their employment, and the vast majority (75%) of all hospital beds in the 4000 hospitals in Mexico are in public institutions, the reality is that many of its poorer citizens, especially those in rural areas, still receive only minimal public care. However, this is improving month after month as *Seguro Popular* builds hospitals and clinics, expands coverage, and enrolls new members. [*See Seguro Popular*]

Until *Seguro Popular* began to insure millions of Mexicans, about half of health-care expenditures in Mexico were out of pocket for private care. This is a reflection of both a preference for private care by an emerging middle class and the fact that some Mexicans—often those in rural areas—simply could not access care within the public system.

Those who are employed by private industry, government or the military are typically given comprehensive coverage—with all medical services being delivered within the public healthcare delivery system—as a benefit of employment. The quality of the treatment facilities and care can vary greatly based on where one resides. This can range from the best-of-class to seriously flawed. Delays for needed treatments in the public system are a common complaint.

In addition to the public system, a thriving private health-delivery system flourishes for those that can afford it, including many private medical practices and private hospitals—most with fewer than two- dozen beds, some with impressive capabilities—and others scarcely more than clinics, without laboratories, radiography equipment or even nurses. [*See Private Hospitals in Mexico*]

And just to make it a bit more complicated, many physicians, including some of the most experienced and highly trained, work both for the public system (which pays a pensions as a benefit) and maintain a private practice.

A Commitment to Continuous Improvement

The Mexican government is in the midst of a long-term crusade to improve quality and reduce inequities in the national healthcare system. This includes a joint effort of public institutions and many private academies, medical association and educational organizations.

The commitment to ongoing improvement is genuine and there are ten overarching efforts currently underway: codes of ethics, quality education, information for and from users for quality improvement, continuous quality improvement processes, incentives, process standardization and monitoring, outcome monitoring, accreditation of institutions and certification of providers, regulation and social participation. While the plan is ambitious, significant measurable improvements are already seen in many of these areas. [*See Welcome to the 4th Edition*]

It is also important to note that one of the goals of the Mexican government is to attract literally millions of retirees from the United States. Mexican officials are well aware of the fact that this will only happen if good-quality healthcare is widely and consistently available and the public's perception is in step with the ever-improving realities of Mexico's vast healthcare system. For those who plan to make Mexico a permanent home, this should be welcome news.

Location, Location, Location

Please remember that there are still many inequities in healthcare delivery in Mexico based on location. Typically, rural areas and southern states are underserved. (This is also true in the United States.) When you hear someone in Guadalajara rave about the care they got in the hospital, do not assume that the same is necessarily going to be true in that far-away coastal fishing village that you fell in love with or a city with a growing population and an aging infrastructure. Be careful when you hear people generalize about all of Mexico when in fact there are huge regionally variations in the availability of service.

Mexico's governmental programs are building new facilities and expanding services all the time, but often the decisions about where to build are going to be based on how a location expands their ability to serve more people. The public agencies are always working on correcting the urban/rural imbalance, but when resources are limited the urban area is understandably more likely to get the hospital and the remote rural area might get visited by a medical team giving vaccinations, doing prenatal checkups and weighing babies once or twice a month.

You also may find that urban clinics and hospitals are utilized beyond the capacity they are designed for in some places. There could be waiting rooms full of people who have waited for hours to see their assigned physician or to get treatment in an emergency room for something non-life threatening. Please note that the number of people being served and thus waiting times may increase on certain days of the week or just after a major holiday.

These and other related factors related to location may enter into your decision between IMSS or *Seguro Popular* or the choice to live in one location or another. The only way to really understand what's best is to go look for yourself and talk to local people about the situation at the hospitals and clinics in their town.

Focusing on the Public System
(IMSS & Seguro Popular)

Like the USA, Mexico has a National Institutes of Health that monitors the health sector and develops and deploys structural reforms in order to increase equitable access to efficient, high-quality health services. Mexico's National Ministry of Health provides healthcare for a significant percentage of the population. Mexico also has a Social Security system that provides benefits including medical care for another large segment of the population.

Here are brief descriptions of the public insurance facets of the Mexican healthcare system. Both IMSS and *Seguro Popular* are available to those expats holding permanent or temporary resident's visa. Those with a visitor's visa may also be treated on an emergency basis, although payment may be expected.

Instituto Mexicano del Seguro Social (IMSS)

An Overview of IMSS

The IMSS is a complex governmental agency providing healthcare and retirement pension benefits for the majority of people employed in Mexico through what is called "involuntary" (mandatory) affiliation. The health plan is paid for through three sources: the government, employers and employees. Non-salaried workers can join through voluntary affiliation for an annual fee of three months' minimum wages (although this is beyond the means of the poorest Mexicans).

IMSS offers a broad range of benefits including emergency treatment, consultations, lab tests, hospitalization, surgery and medications. However, all treatment is given by IMSS personnel and within IMSS hospitals and clinics only.

Patients are assigned a primary care physician who can order testing, refer patients to specialists or to other, larger specialty facilities within the system or recommend hospitalization if needed. It is not unusual for patients to be required to travel, sometimes to Mexico City, sometimes by ambulance, to receive treatment by a specialist.

IMSS runs clinics and hospitals that offer excellent care but the facilities are institutionally functional and rather minimalistic. With rare exception, staff speaks only Spanish and you may need to bring someone with you to help with translation if you don't speak Spanish. Procedures are efficient, but designed to facilitate the treatment of many people with already stretched resources and staffing.

There are significant regional differences in waiting times, availability of blood and medications and you may end up paying for items that aren't available. You may eventually be reimbursed for those that are authorized by IMSS, but that may be an involved process. For routine doctor's visits, appointments are typically made in advance, although long wait times are not unusual. For some locations, appointments are made by phone. At others, you will need to visit the facility to make an appointment. It is best to arrive early because even with an appointment there is the tendency to call patients on a first come, first serve basis.

Hospital staffs are extremely hardworking but Mexican culture assumes you will have a family member with you to assist with personal care tasks: bedpans, bathing and feeding patients when needed and even running errands and performing *tramites* or bureaucratic functions such as pursuing doctors for signatures, standing in line at the pharmacy, picking up lab results, etc. [*See If You Are Hospitalized*]

While it is difficult to evaluate such a large, multi-faceted institution on the basis of the experience of individual users, it is fair to say that IMSS has both its supporters and its detractors. In many ways it is similar to HMOs in the US, with similar limitations and drawbacks. However, the coverage is comprehensive for Mexicans at any age [*See Exclusions and Limitations for Foreigners Applying for IMSS*] and the price is fair.

Foreigners Can Apply for IMSS

IMSS health benefits (but not social services) are available to foreigners who hold temporary or permanent resident visas (formerly FM2, FM3) through application for "voluntary" coverage (as opposed to the mandatory participation through employment). The cost, per person, is based upon age and averages about $350 USD per year. There is no maximum age, however, pre-existing conditions are not covered and there are waiting periods for many specified conditions, so that full coverage is not effective for the first two years.

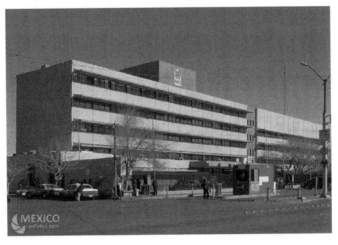

IMSS Hospital in Ciudad Juárez. -Photo by Javier de la Mora

In order to apply you will need a valid temporary or permanent resident visa, passport, birth certificate (translated into Spanish), if married, a marriage certificate (translated into Spanish), proof of residency such as a lease or a phone bill and a completed application and questionnaire forms. Bring multiple copies of these documents along with two photos of yourself (infantile size).

You can apply at the nearest IMSS clinic or hospital. While it is possible to complete this process yourself, if you do not speak Spanish you may want to hire a bi-lingual speaker who specializes in facilitating the process for foreigners. Once the paper and signatures are obtained at the nearest IMSS medical facility, you will need to take them to an IMSS office and when they are accepted, you will need to make payment at a bank and the receipt has to be submitted back to the IMSS office in order to obtain your IMSS card.

Once you have your IMSS identification booklet (*carnet*), you will need to bring it to appointments along with validation of premium payment. For those purchasing their own IMSS, coverage must be renewed annually without the requirement of showing birth and marriage certificates. Foreign visitors to Mexico can use IMSS hospitals for emergencies only, however you would need to be prepared to pay for services with cash just as you would do in a private hospital in Mexico. They will not take insurance and probably won't take credit.

Please note that local procedures may vary, but this is the standard.

Exclusions and Limitations for Foreigners Applying for IMSS

Pre-existing conditions are excluded from benefit coverage (permanently, although this is something you can discuss with your IMSS physician), but do not exclude treatment for other illnesses that began during your stay in Mexico. You must let IMSS doctors know about pre-existing conditions or your coverage may be cancelled and denied in the future. Pre-existing illnesses are defined as:

- Chronic degenerative disease such as that which is seen with long-standing diabetes, liver disease (cirrhosis, hepatitis, etc.), kidney disease (renal failure or renal insufficiency), heart disease (previous heart attack, arrhythmia, or alular disease), lung disease (chronic bronchitis, emphysema, etc.), neurological disease (multiple), cerebrovascular disease (stroke or TIA), peripheral vascular disease, and many others.
- Drug or alcohol dependency
- History of traumatic or muscular injury that continues to require treatment
- HIV positive status or history of AIDS
- Malignant tumors (cancer)
- Psychiatric illness

Exclusions for the following have time limitations—after which they are covered:

- Benign breast tumors in the first six months after acceptance
- Births in the first ten months after acceptance

The following procedures are excluded in the first year after acceptance:

- Lithotripsy for kidney stones
- Surgery for gynecologic conditions except for cancer
- Surgery for vein disorders

- Surgical procedures for the sinuses, nose, hemorrhoids, rectal fistulas, tonsils and adenoids, hernias (except for herniated spinal discs), and other operations that are also considered "elective," rather than required.
- Surgery for orthopedic conditions are not covered for the first two years after acceptance, nor will IMSS insurance cover these:
- Aesthetic or plastic surgery
- Contact lenses
- Dental care (except for extractions)
- Eyeglasses
- Hearing aids
- Infertility treatments
- Laic surgery or the equivalent
- Preventive care
- The surgical correction of astigmatism
- Treatment of self-inflicted injury
- Treatments for behavioral or psychiatric disturbances

Seguro Popular, Secretaría de Salud (SSA)

An Overview of Seguro Popular

Seguro Popular is public health insurance offered and operated by the National Ministry of Health. Unlike IMSS, which is mandated for employed people, affiliation with the *Seguro Popular* system is voluntary. With hundreds of hospitals and thousands of clinics scattered across both urban and rural Mexico, and with millions of participants, *Seguro Popular* covers most of those not covered under the Social Security program (IMSS). This includes those who are agricultural workers or those who are self employed or unemployed and their families. *Seguro Popular* helped to close the gap between coverage rates for indigenous and non-indigenous people and is now working to close the gap between rural and urban populations.

Seguro Popular is available to those foreigners who have a resident's visa (permanent or temporary). There is no age limit and pre-existing conditions are covered (to the extent that those are covered conditions). The cost is based on an initial interview asking questions to determine your standard of living (Do you have indoor plumbing? Do you own a car? etc.) and the cost is typically very modest. The are no co-pays for affiliates.

What Seguro Popular Covers

While *Seguro Popular* covers a wide range of services, it should be noted that technically *Seguro Popular* is not comprehensive insurance (although I have yet to hear anyone complain about being turned away from treatment, including major surgery such as a joint replacement.) However, please keep in mind that eligible treatments are limited to those on the current list of "interventions."[6] For example, *Seguro Popular* does not cover dialysis, but will cover many of the medications associated with dialysis and renal failure.

The *Seguro Popular* program has grown significantly since first offered in 2002. At that time there were only 78 covered interventions in total and those were primarily things like screening for breast cancer and diabetes, pre-natal care and well-baby care (vaccinations). As of 2016, *Seguro Popular* clinics and hospitals diagnosis and treat 287 conditions, have approved 647 medications and supplies for coverage and cover 149 conditions that require surgery or major medical interventions.

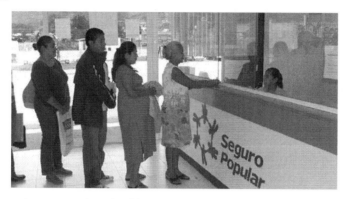

Just over a decade old, *Seguro Popular's* facilities are new

So, while not completely comprehensive, coverage is extensive and has continuously improved over the years. Medicines are typically generic and supplies of prescribed medicines sometimes run short. You may need to rely on a family member to purchase medications at a commercial pharmacy and payment may be reimbursed if it is a medication from the covered list.

In addition to expanding coverage, *Seguro Popular* has been building hospitals and clinics to make healthcare more widely available. However, treatment facilities are limited to those managed by the Ministry of Health and treatment by private hospitals or private medical practices will not be covered. If you are covered by *Seguro Popular* and you are traveling within Mexico, you can be treated at any facility operated by the Ministry of Health. Typically, you will not see the same doctor every visit, although if you are being treated by a specialist, you may. However, this is not guaranteed.

CAPASITS Clinics for HIV/AIDS

Seguro Popular covers HIV/AIDS (called *VIH* in Mexico) treatment (IMSS does not for foreigners) through special clinics called CAPASITS (*El Centro Ambulatorio para la Prevención y Atención en SIDA e Infecciones de Transmisión Sexual*).

This treatment includes antiviral treatment. At the time of this writing, antivirals *Efavirenz*, *Tenofovir* and *Emtribitavina* are typically available, *Atripla* is not. The availability may vary from time to time, or regionally. However, the cost is free for HIV and AIDS treatment and all public care is low cost as it is considered a human right. In Mexico, HIV/AIDS affects the young (especially teens) and poor disproportionately. [*See Sexually Transmitted Infections*]

Applying for Seguro Popular

Seguro Popular is administered through the *Hospitales Generales* by the National Ministry of Health. Application is made at a local *Seguro Popular* hospital (or Ministry of Health clinic where there is no hospital.) There are hospitals in many cities. As a foreign national applying for *Seguro Popular*, you will need to bring your passport, visa residency card (green card), CURP verification, a utility bill to verify your address and a birth certificate that has been an apostiled.[7] [*See CURP and INAPAM Program*] National and naturalized residents are required to submit a birth certificate and voter card. It is recommended that you bring both original and photocopies. Photos are not necessary. If you do not speak Spanish, you will need to bring a Spanish speaker with you. Do not expect anyone to speak English!

Except in an emergency, do not expect to walk in to be treated at a *Hospital Generales*. You must be referred by the medical staff at a clinic run by *Seguro Popular*. It is unlikely that you will find anyone who speaks English at a clinic. You will need to bring a Spanish speaker with you in in nearly all instances.

Most *Seguro Popular*'s provide their own ambulance service, but you should verify this with your local hospital. You will need to bring your family's *Seguro Popular* ID card with you and typically Mexicans bring their own *mica* (plastic envelope) for storing medical records to clinic and hospital visits. [*See If You Are Hospitalized*] Although the card issued by *Seguro Popular* is a smart card with a chip that stores vital data for your whole family with each visit, you are still likely to accumulate paperwork.

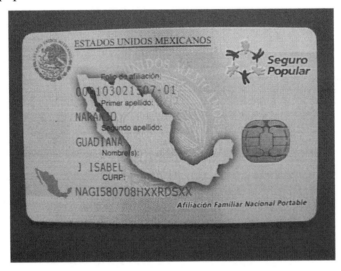

Seguro Popular family smart card with electronic chip

Managing Your Expectations

Public hospitals to not provide the same level of nursing care you expect in the USA or Canada. This is not neglect or malpractice. You are in a different culture where family members are expected to provide nearly all personal care are such as feeding, bathing and toileting. You may be expected to provide your own bedding: blankets and sheets, although pillows may not be permitted at all. Of course, you will need to brings your own toiletries and I have always found a package of baby wipes to be indispensable.

It is vitally important that you plan for the reality of being hospitalized if you are going to be covered under the public system in Mexico. [*See If You Are Hospitalized*] Unless you are in isolation for an infectious disease, you will be staying in a ward with others being treated for similar complaints (heart, liver, orthopedics, etc., although men and women are in separate wards. Children have their own treatment areas and are not allowed to visit adults. Privacy and space is minimal and at night family members may be allowed to sleep on the floor. Electronics other than an inexpensive cell phone may not be allowed or safe and even charging a cell phone may not be permitted. There are no bedside phones or televisions, although small radios may be tolerated if played softly.

Quality of Care

Despite the restrictions and the lack of amenities and personal services, the medical care in Mexico is universally good to excellent and *Seguro Popular* is no exception. The differences tend to be cultural and the fact that Mexico is a developing country providing care for millions of people. The decisions they make reflect the need to provide the best care they can for as many people as possible. The public health sector in Mexico generously provides quality care even for those of us who are not citizens and it is widely considered to be among the best healthcare in the world.

Renewals & Information

After application, *Seguro Popular* is valid for 6 months or until one has had the physical. After the physical, it is valid for 3 years. After this period, one must reapply. Information about *Seguro Popular* can be obtained 24 hours a day, 365 days a year at 01 800 7-8527.[8]

Other Government Programs

Instituto de Seguridad y Servicios Sociales para los Trabajadores del Estado (ISSSTE) covers only government employees. *Secretaría de Defensa Nacional*, *Secretaría de Marina* and *Petróleos Mexicanos* (Pemex) have their own health programs, which cover military and naval personnel, and petroleum workers, respectively.

Blended Solutions

If you are considering retirement or residency in Mexico, you may want to consider blending IMSS or *Seguro Popular* coverage with other healthcare options such as Medicare, private insurance, a clinic/HMO plan, air evacuation insurance or by simply paying out of pocket for private care. In other words, for some foreigners IMSS or *Seguro Popular* functions essentially as major medical insurance and they rely on private physicians for routine care. Please note that it is not possible to have both IMSS and *Seguro Popular* coverage.

Remember that there is no IMSS coverage for pre-existing conditions and there is a two-year waiting period for full coverage, so you will need additional coverage at least for that timeframe. Also, it is not clear how long IMSS benefits will be available to foreigners given that the system is already operating beyond capacity. "The system is saturated, that's the reality of it," says Juan José González, a spokesperson for the IMG regional office in Guadalajara, Mexico's second largest city.

There is also the possibility that public benefits for foreigners—especially those of *Seguro Popular* and those IMSS benefits that are not associated with family ties or employment—are subject to political scrutiny, especially if terms between the USA and Mexico become strained over issues such as who pays for building a wall.

CURP and INAPAM Program

The CURP is universal registration number (and identification card) that identifies every person who lives in Mexico, both Mexicans and foreigners, CURP (*clave única de registro de población*.)[9] It can be obtained at a *Registro Civil* office, however your resident's visa and passport will be required. However, as with all *trámites* (bureaucratic procedures) in Mexico, it is a good idea to also bring copies of your *Comprobante de domicilio* (proof of address as a lease or utility bill), birth certificate and copies of your visa and passport. You should have the flimsy document you are given laminated. You can obtain additional copies online.[10]

If you are age 60 or older, and you have your CURP card in hand, you may want to apply for an INAPAM program card as well. With this card you may qualify for a wide variety of senior discounts (typically 5%) on everything from transportation to pharmaceuticals. It is relatively easy to apply and the benefits add up. You will need to bring your original visa, CURP card, passport and proof of address. You will be asked to complete a document with about 30 questions in Spanish, so if you don't speak Spanish, bring a bilingual friend or family member. They will take your photo for the ID (or send you to a nearby photographer) and you will be fingerprinted for the card. Remember to use it once you have it.

The Red Cross in Mexico

Like most places in the world, the Red Cross in Mexico (Cruz Roja Mexicana), provides assistance during major disasters such a floods and hurricanes. However, that is where the similarity ends. The Red Cross in Mexico offers far more extensive services that are unrelated to public disasters such as ambulance services, emergency first aid, soliciting blood donations and hospital care in a system of hospitals that it funds and controls.

The Red Cross in Mexico is typically the first responder in the case of auto accidents or on the scene after the commission of a crime. Even more surprising: Red Cross in Mexico is not affiliated with the International Red Cross and it is entirely funded by private donations.

Both the Red Cross and the Mexican National Health Service (IMSS) have hospitals in all major cities in Mexico—in addition to various private hospitals. Some cities have municipal hospitals or general hospitals managed by *Seguro Popular* as well. While the IMSS hospitals primarily provide care only for Mexicans and expats who are employed or who can afford to pay premiums, and not every *pueblo* (town or village) has a *Seguro Popular* Hospital, those who are not covered must rely on either a municipal or Red Cross hospital for care—where hospital services are either free or charged on a sliding scale. (IMSS hospitals will treat visitors in an emergency but will not accept other insurance.) Emergency care in cities is typically good to excellent.

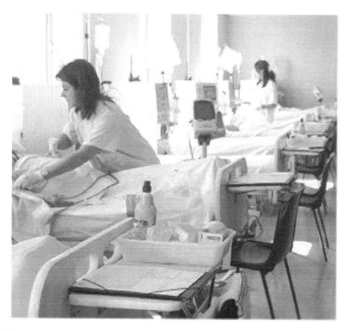

The Cruz Roja provides vital services such as dialysis across Mexico

Outside of the cities, in the many small *pueblos* that dot the countryside, in-hospital emergency care is often simply not available. People in these cases are totally dependent on the Red Cross to provide emergency care. The normal procedure is to transport emergency patients to the nearest hospital by ambulance—typically in the nearest city.

Funds for the Red Cross in Mexico are raised by groups of volunteers who are visible in the streets asking for handouts and solvency is always an issue. Because of the Red Cross' importance in providing a safety net for so many people, and their chronic and urgent need, it is important to help them in whatever way you can. They are responsible for saving many lives and if you were ever in an emergency situation in Mexico, it is entirely possible that they could help you or a loved one someday.

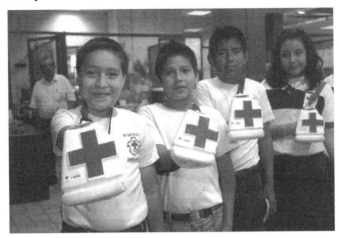

Your contribution provides emergency services throughout Mexico

Licensing of Medical Professionals

Upon fulfilling the requirements to practice as a professional in Mexico, one obtains a *cedula* or license. This is true of both medical doctors and dentists as well as other professions where a license is required to practice including architects, accountants, attorneys, engineers, etc. This certificate is issued by the government and professionals must display this document. If a physician has completed studies in a specialization, they will have a *cedula* to certify them as a general practitioner, and one for each of the specialties that they are legally certified to practice. You can discover if a doctor has a current *cedula* by entering information on the government website.[11]

A *cedula* is different from medical board certification which is more likely to assure that the practitioner you are working with is both certified and competent. [*See Appendix C: Medical Specialties & Medical Boards*]

Medical Board Certification & Medical Specialties

After completing medical school and being awarded a *cedula* (license) to practice by the government, many physicians specialize in some area of medicine. [*See Medical Training in Mexico*]

In many developed countries we rely on various medical boards to certify doctors in medical specialties. This is true in Mexico as well. In Mexico there are a many medical associations, medical boards, credential-granting organizations and governmental and non-governmental agencies that evaluate medical qualifications. [*See Appendix C: Medical Specialties & Medical Boards*]

Medical boards in Mexico are known as *Consejos* and many physicians have been certified in some area of specialization. This means that they are both legally enabled to practice that specialty, they have fulfilled the *Consejos's* training requirements and have passed exams to demonstrate both knowledge and skill in that area of specialization. In order to maintain their board certification, most *Consejos* require continuing education and award credit for publishing, attending conferences and meeting, etc

Although this is a wonderful trend in Mexican medicine, current lack of certification should not necessarily disqualify an otherwise potentially good candidate. There are highly trained, successful physicians that are not certified by any board and many good hospitals lack accreditation as well. [*See Accreditation of Hospitals*] However, those medical professionals who have been board certified should be considered well qualified.

A Good Source of Medical Referrals

Beyond the value of knowing which physicians are board certified, you may find that these various associations and boards can provide an excellent place to find a good physician referral, especially if you are seeking a medical specialist. While some may not show membership information online, most of them do. If you don't find what you need online, contact the organization and provide them with your location, they may be able to direct you to their nearest members. However most have some sort of membership list or search feature that allows you to located local physicians.

Most of these websites are in Spanish, however you can use online tools to help you translate in order to find the information you need. [*See Helpful & Potentially Lifesaving Language Tips*]

Chiropractics & Homeopathy

If you are from the United States, you may consider Chiropractics (*Quiropráctica*) or Homeopathy (*Homeopátia*) to be questionable medical approaches or simply "alternative" practices and outside the mainstream.

This is not true in much of the world, and it certainly isn't true in Mexico where you will find Chiropractic and Homeopathic physicians receive high regard (although only MDs are allowed to practice medicine in Mexico). In Mexico you will frequently see *consultarios* for Chiropractors and Homeopaths on city streets.

Homeopathy has been practiced in Mexico since 1850 and you will often find you can receive treatment in conjunction with Homeopathic pharmacies. A few pharmacies manufacture homeopathic medicines, and many pharmacies sell remedies to doctors and patients alike.

There are two official schools that offer training as a medical doctor and homeopath: the *Polytechnic Institute* and the *Escuela Libre*, both in Mexico City. Several other schools including *La Escuela Nacional de Medicina y Homeopátia* in Mexico City, *El Instituto Superior de Medicina Homeopática de Enseñanza e Investigación de Monterrey* in Nuevo León and the *Instituto de Estudios Tecnológicos y Superiores de Tepic Nayarit* offer postgraduate education for medical doctors.

If you are in Mexico and you are suffering from any condition that has not responded to traditional treatment, you may want to consider trying the Chiropractic or Homeopathic options. After all, you will find rates are very reasonable, both approaches tend to support other forms of treatment and neither is invasive or toxic.

Embassies & Consulates in Mexico

Getting Help from Embassies & Consulates

While each country will only have one Ambassador and Embassy in Mexico City, the seat of the Mexican federal government, there may be many Consulates (offices) with various officials (Consulars) and their staffs that work to represent their country of origin and its citizens in a foreign land. Consulates are essentially branch offices for Embassies.

These offices perform many duties that may be required by travelers and Expats. For example, they typically can help with lost or stolen passports. A U.S. Consular Officer can also assist in locating appropriate medical services, as well as in notifying friends, family or employers of an emergency.

In fact, the US and Canadian Embassies in Mexico maintains a database of physicians who speak English, and who are recommended by them based upon their having rendered satisfactory services to American personnel in the past as well as having provided the Embassy with details of their medical training and experience.

You will notice that the physicians on the embassy lists are located in Mexico City (DF, or Distrito Federal). This is because the embassies are located in Mexico City (as are the majority of expatriates). However, this is not the only source of help.

American Embassy & Consulate in Mexico City

Paseo de la Reforma 305
Colonia Cuahtemoc 06500
Mexico DF
Telephone: +52 55 5209 9100
If you are calling from within Mexico City, just dial 5209 9100
The US Embassy in Mexico Website[12]

Canadian Embassy & Consulate in Mexico City

Schiller 529
Colonia Rincon del Bosque
Polanco 11560
Mexico DF
Telephone: +52 55 5724 7900
If you are calling from within Mexico City, just dial 5724 7900
The Canadian Embassy in Mexico Website[13]

British Embassy & Consulate in Mexico City

Río Lerma 71
Col Cuauhtémoc
06500 México DF
Telephone: +52 55 1670 3200
If you are calling from within Mexico City, just dial 1670 3200.
The British Embassy in Mexico Website[14]

Consulates are Outside of Mexico City

If you are outside of Mexico City and you become seriously ill, consular officers—at many consulate offices scattered throughout Mexico—can also assist in finding a local doctor or hospital and in notifying your family and friends about your condition. Consulates can also help arrange the transfer of emergency funds to you if you become destitute as a result of robbery, accident, or other emergency. For a list of US, Canadian and UK consulates in Mexico [*See Appendix D: USA, Canadian & UK Consulates in Mexico*]

While this guide is focused on the needs of English speakers, primarily those from the US, Canada and the United Kingdom, citizens from many other countries may be able to locate their own county's consulates within Mexico. Embassy World provides an online searchable database to help you locate yours. If you need to contact a Mexican Embassy in your home country, you may be able to locate them in this directory.

The US Embassy Physician List

This is a list of physicians that the US Embassy in Mexico City (where the Embassy is located) refers people to. It is organized by medical specialty. All the physicians here have some level of English skill, have provided background information and performed satisfactory service in the past.

If you are outside of Mexico City and want a referral to a local physician or hospital from the US Embassy, contact the nearest US Consulate in Mexico. [*See Appendix D: USA, Canadian & UK Consulates in Mexico*]

While the US Embassy does not guarantee the skill or qualifications of theses doctors, at least communication in English should be possible and it might be assumed that if they received complaints about a physician the embassy would remove them from the list. This is one of the reasons it is important to register complaints if you have issues with your treatment. [*See Complaints About Medical Care*]

Pharmacies & Medicines in Mexico

An Overview of Mexico's Pharmacies

When you spend any time in Mexico, it soon becomes clear that there are a lot of pharmacies here. In a city you may find more than one on a block, perhaps even three or four. Even in the countryside, there will typically be several pharmacies in a small town. They may even have one that is open for 24 hours, although you may have to bang on the door at four in the morning to wake the pharmacist up.

Most medications, with the exception of narcotics, antibiotics, and pseudoephedrine (a common ingredient in cold medicines) are available without a prescription and you can have a taxi driver pick up medications and deliver them to you if you are too ill to go yourself.

There are basically two kinds of *farmacias*: those that are allowed to dispense prescribed narcotics and those that are not. By far the overwhelming numbers are the later group. And these will vary from the tiniest storefront with a little counter and one pharmacist to Sanborns, the upscale pharmacy with departments selling everything from boxes of candy to clothing, magazines and the latest music CDs. You'll find them in most cities.

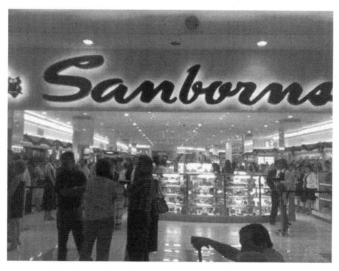

The Sanborns in Mexico City has 2,684,088 "likes" on their Facebook page

Many pharmacies have medical consultorios situated next door where, for 25 or 30 pesos, you can have a (typically) fresh-out-of-medical-school doctor look at your throat, take your temperature, check your blood pressure and write you several prescriptions that you can have filled for a few dollars at the pharmacy. In fact, there is an industry phenomenon in Mexico—generic medications—sold by a chain of pharmacies knows as *"Farmacias Similares."* Their mascot, often found dancing to upbeat music in an over-sized costume, is "Doctor Simi," a familiar figure who is either loved or loathed by passers-by.

There's an App for That!

There's a fast, easy way to find nearby medical treatment and pharmacies in Mexico: Use your cell phone. The Mexican *Secretaria de Salud* (Secretary of Health) provides free downloadable apps for Android (4.1 and up) and OSi cell phones. These apps provide information about the locations and distance to over 5000 hospitals, pharmacies and medical offices. The apps, called RadarCiSalud, can be downloaded from Google (for Android) or iTunes for iPhone, iPad or Apple Watch.[15],[16]

Why So Many Pharmacies?

In Mexico, it is common for people to consult a pharmacist when they are ill before they see a private physician, partly because pharmacists do dispense based on their own evaluation or because the patient wants a certain medicine, and partly because the pharmacist is free or the affiliated *consultorio* is low cost, making it affordable to people with limited incomes. Also, a visit to a nearby *farmacia* is fast, whereas a visit to a doctor at a public health clinic may take hours and precious time away from work.

Reliance on medications is a long-standing tradition in Mexico. When the Spaniards arrived, there was already a vast body of knowledge about medicinal plants among the indigenous peoples here. The Aztecs identified and used about 400 different herbal remedies and recorded many of these in their codices, book-like written and illustrated records. This tradition continues both in the sense that many of these remedies are still used in the countryside and it is common to find people selling herbs as remedies in the local marketplaces—and in wide proliferation of the modern-day *farmacia*.

Of course, the dark side of this tradition is that the easy access to medications leads to self-diagnosis and self-prescribing with the erratic results you might expect. I recently visited a friend who was hospitalized by a physician after he had received "treatments" at a pharmacy-affiliated *consultorio* for the following infections: eye, stomach, throat, diarrhea, jock itch and what seemed to be a serious inflammation of the leg. When he finally was seen by a private physician, more dead than alive, he was immediately hospitalized where he remained for five days for a life-threatening thrombosis, followed by nearly two months of bed rest.

So the lesson is: for anything more serious than a sneeze or a bug bite, it's a good idea to see a physician who isn't working for a pharmacy. But it's great to have a place where you can get your blood pressure checked, to take the kids when they have a cold and ask all the questions you want for a few pesos.

The Quality of Mexican-Manufactured Pharmaceuticals

Medicines manufactured in Mexico are widely regarded as of high quality. The Mexican Health Ministry, a powerful government agency, oversees the manufacturing and sales of Mexican produced drugs. Mexican manufactured pharmaceuticals are exported to other countries including the US where they are often packaged and sold as brand-name drugs.

All Mexican manufactured drugs— both brand name and generic— are made to the same high standard and from the same high-quality materials. However, you should be aware that not all drugs sold in Mexico are manufactured there, and those made in China or other Asian countries do not fall under the same government supervision as those that are Mexican made.

A recent post made anonymously by an industry insider had this insight about Mexican-manufactured pharmaceuticals:

> "I work for a Mexican pharmaceutical company (not a very large one, family owned). We manufacture a couple of drugs under license, but mostly generics. Most people in the US don't believe me, but we sell some of our products to one of the Top 10 pharmaceutical companies in the US (let's call it BigPharmaX). Said company sells them under their own brand name in the US."

> "We sell each piece to BigPharmaX at about $7 Mexican Pesos, which is currently about $0.45 USD. Still very profitable for us. We even print their branded packaging locally."

> "I don't know much about the supply chain in the US and their markups, but you can find our product, sold by the BigPharmaX company brand label with a price of about $40 USD in most major American drugstores. In the back, of course, it says "Made in Mexico"."

> "The same exact product you will find, under a different brand name, made by the same factory, in any major Mexican pharmacy for not more than $40 Mexican Pesos (about $2.50 USD)."

> "We use top-of-the-line German and Dutch machines, and the raw materials and excipients are from Germany, Switzerland, South Korea, Mexico, or Japan. Only one a few of our products use Chinese raw materials, but we have very strict quality control procedures in place and still use quality excipients like BASF (which I'm told is very important for achieving the right timing in Extended Release and similar formulations). Also, for example, the glass vial we use for injectables has a proprietary formulation with enhanced UV filtering in UV sensitive formulations, that we developed and have manufactured to our specification. I'm pretty sure I can say our quality is the best, we don't cut corners. For comparison the leading European lab doesn't use UV filtering glass in the same products, trusting the cardboard box and shortening expiry dates."

> "We hire a fancy European firm for quality auditing and assessment in order to get a certificate each year. Each year they they leave impressed with our commitment to quality."

Finding Your Medicine in Mexico

I was recently asked by a couple considering moving to Mexico whether a life-saving US-manufactured drug will be available here, and what the local brand name of the drug would be. It's not an uncommon question: many people considering Mexico as a place to live often ask whether they can get their medicines locally.

The answer in an overwhelming number of situations is "yes," although discovering what that medicine is called here, and if it is the exact same brand, or chemically the same as the brand you take in your home country, will require some investigation.

Here are some suggestions that may help.

Drugs are marketed under different names in different countries, but the chemical name of the medicine you are taking should not vary. You can find out what the chemical name is from your pharmacist and/or the information fact sheet that the drug is shipped with.

One of the best ways to make certain your usual drug and a Mexican drug are the same is to look at the chemical diagram on the information sheet. If they are exactly the same, then it is the same chemical, although the dosage and form (e.g. number of mg and capsule vs. pill) may be different. The Internet Drug Index is an online resource that may be able to help you identify the Mexican manufacturer for a specific medication.[17]

Another way to find a Mexican source is to contact the manufacturer of your pharmaceutical and ask them if the specific drug you need is distributed in Mexico. If it is, ask what name it trades under here. If they don't distribute in Mexico directly, ask if they have a Mexican affiliate, as oftentimes a foreign company wishing to operate in Mexico must open a separate business here to trade regulated products.

If the drug is distributed under license in Mexico, contact the Mexican company and ask them about the medicine you are looking for. Ask using the generic chemical name, not the brand name. If they do have it, ask what name it trades under in Mexico and where it is distributed.

Another way to find out the name of your medicine is to ask a pharmacist in Mexico. While there are many *farmacias* here, not all pharmacies are the same. If you are looking for US, Canadian or European drugs or their Mexican equivalent in Mexico, you are most likely to find them in larger pharmacy chains and stores like Sanborns.

In the unlikely event that you are not able to find your specific medication—either your home-country brand or a chemical equivalent—you always have the option of bringing a supply with you (***this does not apply to narcotics or psychotropic drugs or cold medicines containing Pseudoephedrine***) along with the prescription and the original container to use temporarily, and seeing a medical specialist in Mexico who can prescribe a new medication for you. Of course, this is essentially starting over with all that implies.

Many of the drugs sold in the US, Canada, and Europe are actually produced in Mexico, and almost every drug (or an equivalent) will be available for your use here. However, in some rare circumstances a specific essential drug you are taking might not be available in Mexico. If so, you will need to discover this before making long-term plans, or if possible, to have that medication dispensed to you by special arrangement.

Pirated Medications

If you spend any time in Mexico, it soon becomes obvious that there are all kinds of pirated (counterfeit) products: music CDs, movies, video games, clothing, etc. Pirated medications have even started showing up in pharmacies. Pirated popular sellers, especially diabetes treatments, but even aspirin have been found primarily in small, independent pharmacies in border towns. Some of these are drugs that are expensive for locals in their authentic form, so small outlaw labs with lax quality control may be packaging generic compounds in counterfeit, lookalike vials, bottle and boxes bearing logos and labels that are designed to deceive the customer.

Legitimate drug manufacturers are organizing to defeat the problem of drug piracy by adding more security features to the packaging, such as holograms, bar codes, and manufacturers' data. As a consumer, you can protect yourself by avoiding drugs being sold significantly below the normal market price in Mexico and purchasing from only a recognized national chain of pharmacies, perhaps one associated with *Asociacion Nacional de Distribuidores de Medinas, A.C.* or *Farmacia Similares*.[18] [*See Farmacias Similares*]

Advertising & Self Medication

Like in the US, widespread advertising of drugs on television has become common. Unfortunately, in a country with a toxic combination of no need for prescriptions for non-controlled drugs (you can obtain many pharmaceuticals other that narcotics and antibiotics without a prescription) and high rates of poverty this can be a problem. Antibiotics, long available without a prescription, currently require one, no doubt because they were improperly administered and generally overused.

When people don't have the money for a doctor, it increases the likelihood of self-medicating leading to overdose, toxic combinations of drugs or simply taking an inappropriate medicine. However, anyone can fall under the spell of advertising and skip seeing the doctor, thus self-medication is a growing problem in Mexico.

Which Type of Pharmacy Do You Need?

Pharmacies come in two classes: those that are allowed to sell controlled or regulated drugs (referred to as *primera clase*) and those that are not, (referred to as *segunda clase*). The majority of pharmacies are *segunda clase*. *Medicinas controladas* (controlled medicines) are those that are most likely to be abused and you cannot purchase them without a prescription from a registered Mexican doctor. Furthermore, pharmacists are tightly regulated by the Sector Salud branch of the federal government of Mexico and anyone caught selling *medicinas contraladas* without prescription is subject to loss of license, fines and even jail.

In the same way that physicians are more accommodating with their ill patients by making home visits, you may find this true of pharmacies as well. Some pharmacies take phone orders of non-controlled medicines and will arrange for a taxi to deliver them to your home if you are ill. It is also possible that even in the countryside a small town may have an overnight pharmacy.

If You Travel to Mexico for Low-Cost Medicines

Although there are people who specifically travel to Mexico—primarily to border towns—to purchase low-cost medications, you should be aware that you must have a valid Mexican prescription in order to purchase controlled medicines. US, Canadian or other foreign prescriptions are not accepted in Mexico.

Bringing controlled substances back into the US or Canada is illegal unless you have the proper authority and is never recommended. [*See The War on Drugs in Mexico*] It is important to declare medicines purchased in Mexico when asked to do so by custom agents and there are limits on the number of doses you can take to most countries. For example, US customs imposes a 50-dose limit.

Unless you live near the border, or need lifesaving medication that is very costly where you live, it is unlikely that you will be able to compensate for travel costs with the lower prices. The People's Guide to Mexico may be able to help you decide.[19]

On the other hand, for those who live in Mexico, most pharmaceuticals are priced well below what you might pay in Europe of other parts of North America and thus offer a tremendous benefit for those who take medicines regularly.

The United States State Department recommends the following for travelers: Carry a letter from your attending physician, describing your medical condition and any prescription medications, including the generic names of prescribed drugs. If you take prescription medication, make sure you have enough to last the duration of the trip, including extra medicine in case you are delayed. Pack your medication in your carry-on bag, since checked baggage is occasionally lost. Always carry your prescriptions in their labeled containers, not in a pill pack.

The War on Drugs in Mexico

For the most part, the War on Drugs in Mexico does not impact visitors nor expats. However, it is important to remember that there is a very active and ongoing war against trafficking illegal drugs. That would include narcotics (heroin, cocaine, opiates), marijuana, and pseudoephedrine (an ingredient used in many cold medications as well as being a sought-after chemical precursor in the illicit manufacture of methamphetamine and methcathinone). Do not bring your cold medicine to Mexico.

Although recent legislation has approved the use of medical marijuana for a very limit spectrum of serious illnesses, buying, selling or possession of marijuana is illegal in most of Mexico. Only a handful of people have been approved for legal treatment. [*See Medical Marijuana*] If you go to a doctor and ask for pain killers, narcotics or medical marijuana it will be assumed that you are seeking recreational drugs even if you have a legitimate health issue. Don't come to Mexico seeking illegal drugs.

Marijuana is not legal in Mexico. Possession of small amounts was de-penalized in Mexico City only. This basically means that a first time offender must participate in a drug rehab program rather than going to jail. However, if you are not a Mexican citizen and you are caught with a joint, it is just as likely that will be charged and given a jail sentence or deported since substance abuse programs are for Mexican nationals. There is no reason the Mexican government should be obligated to rehabilitate non-citizens.

This is serious business. Consider that people are dying in the war on drugs for trafficking in Mexico. Consider that an American woman, a tourist, was detained in Mexico in 2016 for attempting to cross the border with Sudafed, a cold medication containing pseudoephedrine, in the original packaging. Medicines containing pseudoephedrine are not allowed in Mexico. That means that Sudafed or other brands of US cold medicines are illegal here. It cost her $1500 in cash to retain an attorney and she was not released by authorities until the U.S. Consulate was able to successfully negotiate on her behalf. Expect zero tolerance.

Farmacias Similares

In Mexico, generic drugs are not just a second, lower-cost drug option. They are the cornerstone of *Farmacias Similares* and an entire private populist medical-delivery system. *Farmacias Similares* is a chain of pharmacies that typically have adjacent, low-cost medical clinics (*Consultorios Medicos*) with doctors who give exams and treat ill patients who walk in off the street. There are no appointments and treatment is on a first-come-first-serve basis.

Farmacias Similares are well known because of widespread advertising and the frequent presence of Dr. Simi, a larger-than-life dancing character that represents the chain in front of many stores to the delight of small children.

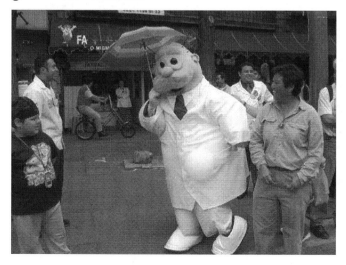

Dancing with Dr. Simi is fun for kids

37

With consultations priced at around $2 USD pesos and the majority of medicines priced at about $5 USD, some level of low-cost medical care is now available to Mexicans who are uninsured or simply cannot take the time to wait for help (nor the time off work) that is often required with public health facilities.

Farmacias Similares are also a reliable source of medical care for the immediate needs of travelers and foreign residents in many situations. However, this is not the place for most emergency treatment or serious or life-threatening situations (unless there are no other options). In emergencies you need to call 911 or the Red Cross for an ambulance.

Most visits to a *Farmacia Similares* will result in being handed several prescriptions that can be filled at the pharmacy next door. (After all, a pharmaceutical company producing generic versions of patented drugs sponsors these clinics.) However, you are not obligated to fill them there, nor to fill all of them at your own discretion.

If you do fill a prescription, do take the medicines as directed. The medicines are typically effective for minor illnesses and the times and dosages are carefully written out for you. Pharmacy-associated medical exams are appropriate for the kinds of everyday illnesses we often experience: colds, flu, stomach complaints, sprains, cuts and abrasions, insect bites and stings, having your blood pressure checked, etc. And, with nearly 4000 *Farmacias Similares* throughout Mexico, you will probably find one nearby.

Accreditation of Hospitals

In the United States and Canada, the accreditation of hospitals and many other healthcare institutions is ubiquitous. You expect your local neighborhood hospital to be accredited and you'd be surprised if it weren't.

In Mexico the situation is different. The whole notion of accreditation is relatively new and very few institutions are. This is not necessarily a reflection of the quality of the facility, staffing, or the care, but simply that the accreditation process is not generally practiced in Mexico. However, this is changing, especially as more international patients visit Mexico as medical tourists.

International Accreditation of Hospitals

The most respected international organization involved in accrediting hospitals is the Joint Commission International (JCI), a division of The Joint Commission, a private, not-for-profit organization dedicated to continuously improving the safety and quality of care provided to the public.

In collaboration with the World Health Organization, the JCI evaluates hospitals accrediting only those that meet high standards in such areas as facilities management, patient safety, medication safety, infection prevention and control.

As of this date there are eight hospitals and one ambulatory care program that have completed the JCI's accreditation process in Mexico. [*See Appendix E: JCI Accredited Hospitals in Mexico*]

Please keep in mind that while accreditation by the JCI is certainly an endorsement of these institutions, not only is this process rigorous—reserved for only world-class institutions, but the JCI moves slowly (as it should) and the notion of accreditation is relatively new within the boundaries of Mexico (let alone international accreditation), thus there are many excellent non-accredited hospitals and teaching institutions in Mexico as well.

Further, the process of obtaining JCI accreditation is very expensive and well beyond the financial reach of many institutions. Even those that have obtain accreditation in the past may elect not to bear the expense of renewal, particularly in a country were few understand its significance.

Private Hospitals in Mexico

There are over 4,000 hospitals in Mexico. Listing them in any meaningful way is very challenging. Assuming that they are all licensed, what criteria do you use? What information is actually useful? For example, if one were to list the "top hospitals" as those affiliated with the best universities, or those with the most beds, or the most prestigious staff, probably 90% of them would be in Mexico City. The same is more or less true for those hospitals with international accreditation. [*See International Accreditation of Hospitals*] And indeed, if you are in need of a top specialists in the country, you will find the majority of them serving at hospitals in Mexico City.

For the individual seeking a local hospital in some other part of the country, the approach discussed above is not helpful. At the back of this book is an appendix with a list with many private hospitals in Mexico. [*See Appendix F: Private Hospitals by State & City*] The criteria for selecting this list is that these are a regionally diverse selection of hospitals that are licensed by the ministry of Health to harvest organs or conduct transplants.

In Mexico, many types of transplants are performed including corneas, bone marrow, stem cell, bone, heart valves, kidneys, liver, heart and lung. There are over 400 hospitals (out of more than 4000 hospitals) located throughout the health sector (social, public and private) that perform different types of transplantation. For a hospital to perform transplants it is required to have a permit issued by the Ministry of Health for that activity, in addition to having trained medical personnel and a well-equipped facility.

Most hospitals that perform transplants are in the capitals of the states and the nation's largest cities. These transplant programs are distinguished by the high levels of surgical skill and the technical capabilities of the hospitals.

The companion book to this one uses another approach to listing private hospitals. In addition to showing listings of reputable hospitals from diverse locations, it lists doctors and hospitals where there are likely to be English-speaking staff. [*See Appendix A: The English Speaker's Guide to Doctors & Hospitals in Mexico*][20]

Medical Training in Mexico

Most medical and dental students in Mexico attend right after high school unlike the USA and Canada where an undergraduate degree is completed first. Remarkably, a free university education is offered to any student in Mexico upon high school graduation provided they are able to pass entrance exams. This free education includes medical, dental and even veterinary school. Public university medical students are required to serve a year in government-supported clinics or hospitals serving remote or disadvantaged communities and is one of the reasons that Mexico is able to offer universal healthcare.

The list of medical schools in Mexico shown in [*See Appendix G: Medical Schools in Mexico*] may prove very useful for you. We know you are probably not going to study medicine, but there are a variety of ways you may use this information.

Medical schools are often using and teaching the most advanced medicine in any country. Often the teachers at medical schools are also in private practice or may have an affiliation with a school's clinical practice.

After completing medical school, a medical student becomes a doctor and can either do a residency in a medical specialty or go straight into a general practice. Admission into a residency program is highly competitive and requires several additional years of low-paying work.

Many medical schools are affiliated with training hospitals or clinics. If you find that a local medical school is affiliated with a hospital where doctors are being trained, it is likely to be a superior hospital. A local medical school may be able provide you with a referral to a newly graduated primary care physician.

The medical schools in Mexico train doctors from all over the world. You are likely to find interns and physicians that speak English as a first or second language through a medical school.

Because of their position at the forefront of current technology and medical practice, consulting with the medical staff at a medical school may help you find exactly the specialists you need so they can be an excellent source of knowledgeable referrals.

Upon graduation and fulfilling government requirements, medical students will be awarded a *cedula* or license to practice. Board certification in a medical specialty requires additional training and meeting additional education requirements. Specialists must also prove their qualifications by passing board examinations called *Exámines del Consejo*. Some doctors in Mexico are certified by both the Mexican medical board in their specialty and the American Academy in that specialty as well. This indicates they have met the stringent training and education criteria required of both the Mexican and the American Academy.

Dentistry in Mexico

Mexico has been a popular destination for medical tourists seeking dental care for a long time. Many of the border towns have dental offices near the crossing that provide more economical solutions for extractions, root canals, bridges, crowns, dentures, implants, orthodontia and cosmetic dentistry. Nearly every small town will have several dentists and you will find hundreds, or even thousands in major cities.

It is not unusual for dental offices in Mexico not to have X-ray equipment so you may be referred to a nearby laboratory for X-rays. This is very routine. However, it is not universally true and there are plenty of dental offices where you'll find X-rays and other state-of-the-art equipment.

I was surprised the first time I went to the dentist and discovered that the clinic was using ultrasound cleaning and intraoral cameras. The dental hygienist at my dentist in Chicago was still scaling teeth with dental instruments and the dentist was still filling teeth with toxic amalgam (now replace in more modern dentistry by resin fillings).

There are thousands of dentists practicing in Mexico, far too many to list here. However, in an appendix at the back of this book is a list of English-speaking dentists who are all in Mexico City. [*See Appendix H: Dental Specialists*] Many are specialist such as Endodontists or Oral Surgeons. If you are seeking a referral to a recommended English-speaking dentist outside of Mexico City, you can contact the nearest consulate for their local recommendations. You can find the consulates listed here: [*See Getting Help from Embassies & Consulates*]. I have also listed many English-speaking dentists in the companion to this book. [*See Appendix A: The English Speaker's Guide to Doctors & Hospitals in Mexico*][21]

Los Algodones and Dental Implants

Los Algodones, Baja California is one of the most unusual places in Mexico, or anywhere in the world for that matter. Located just across the U.S. border, about eight miles west of Yuma, Arizona, this small town with a population of just over 5,400 plays hosts to tens of thousands of visitors from the USA and Canada every year.

While Los Algodones has some of the things you might expect from any border town in Mexico—vendors in open air markets selling souvenirs, sunshine, music, outdoor cafes—what you may not expect are the literally hundreds of dentists, doctors, opticians and pharmacies that line the streets. Many claim that there are more dentists in the four blocks square of *el centro* of Los Algodones than in any other four blocks in the world. There are so many dentists tucked into every corner that they defy counting.

Snowbirds (migratory retirees) and citizens from both Canada and the U.S. flock to Los Algodones for inexpensive dental care, medicines, eyeglasses, and medical care. [*See Medical Tourism*] For many, a trip to Los Algodones is an annual ritual. And why not? Dental procedures are a fraction (typically 25-35% percent) of what they cost on the U.S. side of the border and most of the dentists and their staff members speak English. The dentists are licensed, some are members of the American Dental Association, some were trained in the U.S. and while the work varies in quality somewhat based on the training and experience of the dentist and the quality of the materials used, it is generally good to excellent.

But the real benefit of a place like Los Algodones is that there are important dental options available to patients that are simply not offered to patients of modest means by dentists to the north, namely: those procedures based on dental implants. Why not? Because these procedures are so expensive in the U.S. and Canada that many dentists never or rarely do dental implants and seldom offer the option to those living on a fixed income. If a single tooth is missing, they offer bridges involving healthy teeth to either side of a missing tooth with an artificial tooth filling the gap. If several teeth are missing they offer "partials" or other dental devices. And if a patient needs all, or nearly all, of their teeth replaced, they may be told they need dentures when better options are available just across the border.

In Mexico the recommended solution in all of these instances is much more likely to be a solution based on dental implants. This is by far the preferred treatment if you qualify. (Diabetics and those with some other health conditions may not qualify.) For example, All-on-Four and All-on-Six solutions, where a full-arc bridge is permanently affixed to four or six dental implants, is a much more satisfactory long-term solution than removable dentures for patients who don't have health issues that might eliminate them as candidates.

From the U.S. side, Los Algodones is most easily reached via the international border at Andrade, California. From Andrade, visitors can park their vehicles for a fee in a Native-American owned lot (no overnight parking) and walk across the border, or simply drive across to Los Algodones.

Traditional Medicine

Traditional healing as practiced since long before the arrival of the Spanish is very much alive today in Mexico. Practicing primarily in rural areas, it is fairly easy to find healers who use various forms of divination and shamanic magic and those who prepare medicines using herbal plants. Please respect that while medicinal plants are used by indigenous Mexicans to make many helpful things—soaps, ointment, mosquito repellent, antibacterial gel, cough syrups and shampoos for example, some medicinal plants are threatened or endangered. While their use as traditional indigenous medicine is recognized in Mexico's constitution as a cultural right of native people, as a non-native please be very careful to only take what you personally will use and appreciate that it is a gift from the Earth and the people of Mexico, not yours to exploit.

Curenderos and Chamanes

A *curandero* (or *curandera* for a female) is a traditional folk healer or *chaman* (shaman) in Hispanic America, who is dedicated to curing physical or spiritual illnesses using traditional medicines and spiritual practices. If you travel to rural Mexico, you will almost always be near someone who practices traditional medicine. It has only been within the last generation that any other kind of treatment option has been available in many parts of Mexico, and in some underserved areas, that is still the case.

When I lived in rural Mexico, the nearest pueblo up the road had been only accessible by horse trail a generation ago. There was no road. If you were so sick that the local healer couldn't resolve the matter, you were put on horseback and would have to ride about twelve kilometers to reach medical help (from a doctor, not a hospital). There is a road now and regular bus service, but the help of a local healer is still likely to be sought first.

Hierberos

Where will you find medicinal plants? They are all around you, however without training you may not be able to identify them. In some parts of Mexico, you may find a traditional *hierberos*, or herbalist who may be willing to guide you into the local countryside to teach you how to identify and collect medicinal plants. A few might be willing to teach you to prepare plants as medicine. However, in most instances they simply collect, cultivate and prepare herbal remedies using traditional methods and if you ask, they may be willing to prepare a remedy for you.

Medicinal Herbs & Plants

When the Europeans arrived in Mexico, they were undoubtedly convinced of their superiority as the conquering army. However, when it came to medicine and an understanding of the human body and how it works, the Aztecs were far more advanced.

As an expat, I recognize and use a few medicinal plants—like aloe and chamomile—that are familiar to me. But if you have an ailment, many native Mexicans, especially in the countryside, will be happy to share a long list of remedies and their preparation with such confidence and conviction that you know their knowledge has been passed down from generation to generation. Discussing home remedies is a great conversation starter since almost everyone and their grandmother can dispense healing advice. It isn't always the best advice, but these are people who have had to rely on themselves and many are a cornucopia of knowledge.

The Aztecs knew the medicinal properties of literally thousands of plants. There are over 3000 medicinal herbs and plants used in Mexico today.[22]

Botánicas

Nearly every *mercado* will have a *botánica* selling a wide variety of herbs, seeds, bark, and flowers with medicinal properties—sometimes along with candles and religious figurines. You'll recognize them by the baskets or bags of what look like sticks or bark and dried flowers hanging from the rafters. The plants are often identified by a card displaying the name of the condition or organ they are typically used to treat. When asked, they can frequently give you some suggested methods of preparation, the most common being as a tea.

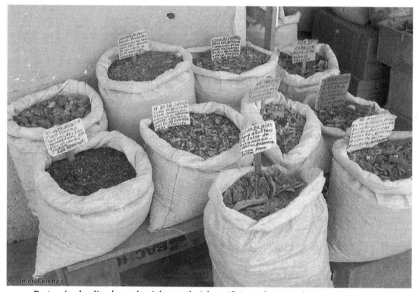
Botanicals displayed with cards identifying the conditions they treat

I recommend that you use moderation when trying any new herbal remedy. I remember that I was so excited when I discovered a wealth of herbs being sold in my local *mercado*, I wanted to make a tea. Not knowing anything about their properties, I opted for a mixture that promised to be a little of everything. I promptly went home, made tea with the mixture and promptly went from feeling just great to feeling a bit green around the gills. I completely underestimated their effect. Nevertheless, when used appropriately, medicinal plants can be helpful remedies. Then again, dosages are not standardized, side effects and contraindications are not given and you proceed at your own risk.

Nearly everyone in Mexico will have a bit of folk wisdom to share to help cure what ails you. If you tell someone you are not feeling well you may find the onslaught of suggestions that follows either helpful or intrusive, wise or outlandish. But the relationship between the people of Mexico and the medicinal plants that live around them has a long, complex and even spiritual history that perhaps we are just beginning to appreciate. So, whether you are told to eat the tail of the scorpion that stung you (personally, I wouldn't), or to sleep bare-backed on a bed of freshly harvested *Cuscuta*, a yellow, leafless parasitic vine pulled from trees for a liver complaint, when it comes to using medicinal plants, use caution and judgment.

Commonly Used Medicinal Plants

Here are a few of the most commonly used medicinal plants and their uses. They are typically considered safe. But that is not a guarantee that they will be appropriate for you.

Aloe Vera

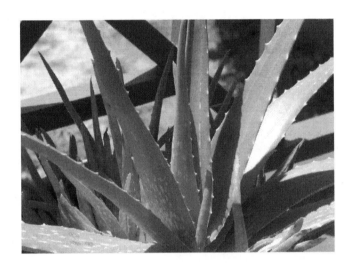

Now known the world over, *aloe vera* is a highly useful succulent species that has been used to treat skin conditions including scrapes and burns, aid the digestive system and to boost the immune system for thousands of years. Aloe has anti-inflammatory, antiseptic, analgesic, and antipyretic properties.

Arnica

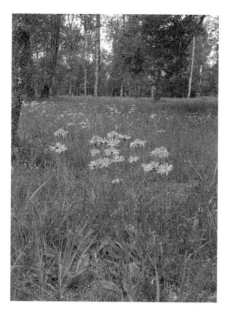

This herbal remedy is applied topically as a lotion or ointment to treat bruises, to reduce swelling and to relieve muscle and bone pain. Ointment made with *arnica* is widely available in *farmacias* and is a popular treatment for children's bumps and bruises.

Gordolobo

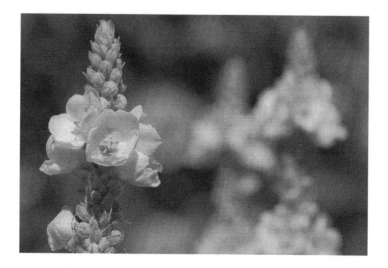

This versatile remedy is prepared as a tea to treat respiratory infections. It has both expectorant properties and is known to inhibit viruses and infections including ear infections. It also stimulates blood flow.

Toronjil

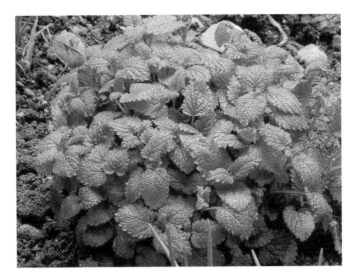

Tea made from *Toronjil* (also known as lemon balm or Melissa), is used to calm the mind and encourage restful sleep. It is also used to boost alertness and sharpen memory and problem solving. It is a powerful antioxidant that supports the liver and the brain and helps to stabilize blood sugar levels and reduce insulin resistance. Toronjil is a popular ingredient in cosmetics because it makes skin look younger.

Valeriana

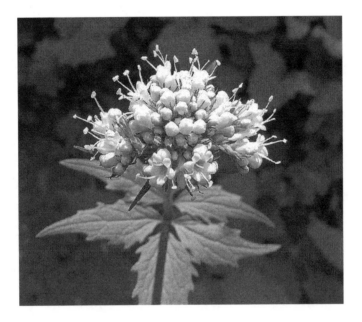

Valeriana is a root that is often used to treat depression, insomnia, and anxiety. Also known for treating muscle spasms and pain, this helpful remedy reduces inflammation, fever and diarrhea, and can be used to disinfect skin wounds.

Nopal & Tunas

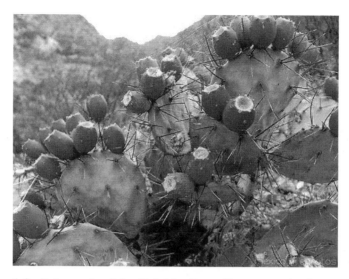

The pads (*nopales*) and fruit (*tunas*) of the Prickly Pear Cactus are both popular food and medicine in Mexico. The spines must be removed from the pads before use and are frequently sold in mercados already de-spined. When the pads are sliced and boiled, they make a vegetable-like dish similar in flavor to green beans—that are used in salads and as a condiment to accompany many dishes.

Highly nutritious, *nopales* are known to lower glucose levels, help with high cholesterol, fight viral infections, and to treat colitis and diarrhea and even to help with hang-overs. A *curendera* even suggested to a friend that he tie the pads to the soles of his feet as a cure. While I don't know how effective they were as medicine, as a food, *nopales* are delicious and their fruits can be peeled and eaten, seeds and all, for a sweet, juicy treat.

Expat Groups for Medical Referrals & Social Networking

The Value of Personal Referrals

There is wide consensus that one of the best ways of finding a good physician is through personal referrals. There is something very reassuring about hearing from someone you trust that a particular doctor is a good one. (However this method may be somewhat over-rated since the referring party may not be qualified to make an evaluation of what's best for you.)

Nevertheless, it is generally helpful to speak to others who know the ropes and referrals are a good place to start your search if you understand you still must make your own evaluations. At least with a personal referral you know that you aren't going to be sent to a doctor the patient didn't like.

But What if You Don't Know Anyone?

But what can you do if you are new in town and don't have any personal contacts that can help you? Or, what if you don't speak Spanish well enough to ask the people around you for a medical referral?

There are many reasons for foreigners to connect with expatriate (expat) communities in Mexico. They can be a source of friendships, work, information, resources (like used furnishings and cars), traveling companions, and of course, medical referrals. You may also find that it is important for your mental health to have at least a few people you can speak to in your native language and who will understand your culture or help you in emergencies.

There Are Times You May Really Need Expat Friends

You should definitely make Mexican friends! But here's why you need a few friendly expats in your circle: The culture of Mexico is of tight-knit families who spend holidays and vacations together. During times of the year like Christmas (*Navidad*) or Easter (*Semana Santa*) virtually all Mexicans go somewhere with their families (even Mexico City becomes a ghost town), and unless you have family connections in Mexico, Mexican friends that include you in their family circle, visitors to your home or expats friends, you might feel very alone.

Making friends with and getting together with other expats can be especially valuable during those times and expat groups often organize social gatherings just to address this need. Remember, you are only human and the holidays are a difficult time for many people, so having people to be with is important for your emotional wellbeing.

If you are invited to join a Mexican family for their festivities, by all means go. It is an honor to be included. But even if you don't, with a little advanced planning, you can have fun. Many expat communities plan parties or other activities at this time to help those of us who might otherwise be alone. It is also a good time to join others in charitable work. Playing Santa, literally in a red suit and beard, in an orphanage in Mexico City, was one of the highlights of my life.

Social Isolation

Social isolation can contribute to two medical problems for expats: untreated depression (sometimes leading to suicide), and alcoholism.

It is estimated that suicide is the 4th leading cause of death for expats from the United States in all countries. USA Today's analysis of State Department statistics — which show only the date and city where a suicide occurred — found that a suicide abroad is reported an average of every two-and-a-half to three days. Every year, Mexico is, by far, the country where more Americans commit suicide than any other. The suicides are typically of young adults and the elderly. In a recent year, 26 American suicides there were reported to the State Department in Mexico. In reality, American suicides abroad are probably much more frequent. The State Department says many American deaths abroad—regardless of cause—are not reported back to the State Department as they should be. Of course, there are many reasons for suicide, but for some, particularly for the elderly, social isolation can be a factor.

This is also true for alcoholism, another serious medical problem affecting some expats. One factor may be that the social life in expat communities in some parts of Mexico is based primarily on partying including hard drinking. Without other options, some expats join in without considering the consequences. Nearly all the large cities in Mexico and those with significant expat populations have regular meetings of Alcoholics Anonymous conducted in English.

Of course, there are better options than making drinking the focus of one's social life, and there are many expats here who actively engage in charity work, teaching, establishing libraries, and sharing their extensive know-how and experience in a plethora of meaningful ways. Connecting with local people who can provide healthy friendships and a sense of community is important and relatively easy to do, particularly if you connect with other expats: many expats friendships start online. You could begin to do this before you move to Mexico so that by the time you arrive you'll be well on your way to integrating into a new community quickly, aware of who is who and what opportunities exist to share and contribute.

Get Involved with a Group Before Moving to Mexico

Rather than wait until you are dealing with an urgent medical need or a dreadful case of loneliness, join and begin to participate in (or at least read) the public communications between members of expat groups as soon as you have identified a few places you might consider living.

Watching and participating in expat communications are excellent ways to begin your initiation into what living in Mexico might offer you. You get to see the day-to-day questions and concerns of members. For example, are they dealing with a lack of water in the public system or merely the lack of horseradish at the *supermercado*?

If You Are Hospitalized

There are other important ways that your expat connections could be critically important to you in Mexico. Because of the tight family relationships in Mexico, it is assumed that there will be family members available to support hospital patients.

By "support" we mean someone from your "family" will be expected to provide the kinds of services you might assume that the nursing staff would perform: feeding, bathing, making the bed, running errands, etc. It would be considered very strange—even tragic—if you did not have someone present with you if you are hospitalized. During a relative's recent hospitalization in a public hospital, I was expected to deliver the used urinals and bedpans to the septic room and the nurse taught me how to bathe my loved one in bed.

In Mexico it is expected that family members will accompany you to the hospital and stay with you in shifts, often spending the night with you, frequently sleeping on the floors in public hospitals, and providing all personal care.

It is important for you, as a foreigner, to have others who would stand-in for your family if you are hospitalized. Even if you have a devoted spouse, they may need relief during a long hospitalization. Ideally you will form an alliance or two with others who can help you and for you to do the same for them. If language is a barrier, having a friend who can translate in an emergency could be life saving.

If you are single, widowed, childless or otherwise alone much of the time, you may want to form a small support group of expats who will act as "family" if one of you is hospitalized. Of course, your Mexican friends might be willing to perform this role as well and potentially you could hire someone. But wouldn't it be better to know this isn't going to be a problem if you become ill?

You May Need Blood Donors

If you are going to have surgery in a public hospital (IMSS or *Seguro Popular*) and there is a likelihood that you will need blood, you will need to provide the blood donors. Typically, this is another function that family members perform in Mexico. But if you do not have family in Mexico, you should arrange a reciprocal arrangement with Mexican friends or other expats in your area.

The donor should go to the hospital, tell the information desk or window that they are donating blood for you and follow the directions they are given. In most cases the blood is banked with that hospital and if you need blood during surgery you will be given blood that has already been tested and prepared, so the donor's blood type does not need to match yours. But a contribution must be made on your behalf.

You may occasionally be called upon through social networks to donate blood to help someone in dire circumstances. It is also not uncommon in Mexico for rare blood types to be in short supply. If you happen to be one with a rare blood type, or you are simply willing to donating blood to help others, giving blood can be a lifesaving gift.

In private hospitals, you do not typically need to provide a blood donor. You will be charged for blood if it is needed as you would any other medical expense.

Types of Expat Groups

Expat groups tend to come in three major categories: those formed around a geographical location (a city or region), those formed around a country of origin (language and culture) and international resources with regional subgroups.

Facebook has many geographical groups in Mexico as well as those that are for the whole country. Some are based on both a location and a language; for example, English speakers in Guadalajara. There are also groups formed around special interests such as nude sunbathing or surfing. For example, Facebooks has a group devoted to English teachers. So, if you have a special interest, make sure to search for it.

The forms that these groups take vary a lot. Some are quite formal with regular meetings, events, newsletters, charitable works, libraries and a dues-paying membership. Others are informal social networks, ideal for finding a friend to go to the movies with or a group to play cribbage or tennis with or to plan a weekend trip to the beach.

The majority of expat groups can be accessed via the Internet. Some are quite active, others seemingly moribund. But remember, the real interactions may not be online but rather in face-to-face meetings or at their events or the action may behind the scenes in email posts back and forth between people who have met as part of the group.

So, whether you connect with a social networking website, user group, email group or blog, register for a few and discover other people who may be as interesting and adventuresome as you are— or as timid and lonely.

Paying for Health Care in Mexico

After concern about the quality and availability of medical care, paying medicals bills, especially for an illness or injury requiring hospitalization, is typically the next most important consideration travelers, expats and retirees have about health care.

Of course there is no single payment option, no one-size-fits-all solution, and you may find that you need several options either at the same time or over time as you make a transition from being a short-term tourist perhaps looking for a place to live, to making longer-term stays in Mexico, then with different needs again if you wish to work in Mexico or if you plan to retire to Mexico on a full- or part-time basis.

So, the objective here is to lay out many of the options you might want to consider and some of the ways that you might want to use them. However, your circumstances are unique and you're the only one who can decide what benefits you must have or what risks you are willing to tolerate.

Like the various payment or insurance options in the United States, Canada or the United Kingdom, these are financial agreements that tend to be complex and full of jargon—made more challenging if the terms are expressed in a language you don't understand.

An appendix at the end of this book attempts to clarify the features and limitations of many of the various types of insurance and benefits in a side-by-side grid to help you compare them more readily. (*See Appendix I: The Insurance Grid*) However, new forms of coverage are being offered all the time, including various types of "gap" insurance designed to cover what other forms of insurance don't cover.

Your Health Insurance from Home

Whether you are a short-term visitor or you establish your residence in Mexico on a longer-term basis, you may be disappointed to learn that your private or employee health insurance from home will probably not cover you in Mexico.

Even if your health insurance does offer coverage outside of your home country, the coverage may be very limited—for example, restricted to emergencies (a good reason for calling an ambulance and entering the hospital through the emergency room) or only accidents or maybe your coverage is limited to just 30 days.

Perhaps your insurance will cover non-emergencies, but the private hospitals in Mexico will most likely not accept an assignment of benefits—even in an emergency—and they will not bill your insurance for you.

In those cases, you would probably have to pay the hospital in cash or with a credit card and submit a claim to your insurance company along with all the bills, receipts, medical records or whatever else they may want in order to authorize reimbursement to you for covered medical expenses. If the hospital bill is in Spanish (and why wouldn't it be), they may require you to have it translated. Giving your credit information to a hospital can sometimes lead to unexpected problems. [*See Not Being Released from the Hospital*]

Even business people who are visiting Mexico as part of their job may be surprised to find that their regular employee health insurance coverage is limited if it exists at all and many private hospitals in Mexico don't take insurance—or only International Health Insurance.

So, whatever your circumstances, it is well worth contacting your Human Resources department or insurance carrier before you leave home and get clarity about what your coverage is, what to do in the event of an emergency or accident and how claims are paid.

Other Medical Insurance Options

Whether you are a traveler, a snowbird spending only part of the year in Mexico, or an expat, there is a bewildering array of medical insurance options—and sorting out what you need from what you don't is a complex and highly personal decision. There are factors such as choosing the type of coverage you want, whether it will be accepted by the institutions where you think you might need it, if pre-existing conditions are covered or not, where the insurance will or won't cover you and of course, the expense of coverage. Another factor to consider is what the potential cost might be if you don't have a particular type of coverage vs. the likelihood of actually using it.

Working with a reputable, licensed, bi-lingual insurance broker who works with insurance carriers on both sides of the USA/Mexico border is highly recommended. (I can personally recommend Tony and Patricia Hamrick with Seguros Insurance.)[23]

Traveler's Insurance

As the name suggests, Traveler's Insurance is designed to provide short-term coverage for the traveler. Travel insurance is intended to cover medical expenses, trip cancellation, lost luggage, flight accident and other losses incurred while traveling, either internationally or within one's own country although benefits and terms will vary. It can be purchased from your neighborhood insurance agent, at airports, or online. You will get the best deal if you purchase it in your home country before you travel.

International Health Insurance

Designed to either provide protection anywhere in the world, or perhaps just a country or two, your international health insurance carrier may also be a good source of medical referrals. Some even have online resources to help members find a doctor or hospital while traveling.[24]

Please keep in mind that while you may have financial coverage for medical and/or hospitalization, that doesn't guarantee that an assignment of benefits will be accepted by every medical facility and hospital. You may still need to pay at the time of service and submit a claim with evidence of payment to the carrier for reimbursement. So, get receipts and copies of itemized bills immediately.

Mexican Health Insurance

If you are living in Mexico on an extended basis, either as an employee, retiree or a self-employed individual, you may want to investigate the many health insurance companies in Mexico that offer medical and hospitalization coverage. Just as in the US and Canada, insurance coverage is often included as a job benefit or available at a greatly reduced monthly premium if you are employed through a large company.

If you are self-employed, investigate purchasing a "group" health insurance plan. These will frequently cover as few as two employees, which could be a husband and wife working together. Individual or family coverage, payable monthly, is widely available throughout Mexico by contacting a broker, through a bank, or directly from the carrier.

The premium rates, the specific losses that are covered or excluded, limits and coverage for pre-existing conditions vary a great deal, and your rate may factor in your age, state of heath, smoking habits, weight, etc. It may be best to work with a bi-lingual broker who can help clarify the policy specifics for you.[25]

Instituto Mexicano del Seguro Social (IMSS)

This is a comprehensive medical and hospitalization insurance available through a government-sponsored program either through one's employment or as a voluntary program participant. It is only available to those who have temporary resident visa *Residente Temporal* or permanent resident visa *Residente Permanente* although there are other restrictions. There is more comprehensive information about the program available in this book in the section on the Mexican healthcare system. [*See Instituto Mexicano del Seguro Social (IMSS)*]

Seguro Popular

This is a Mexican public health program offering a wide range of medical care and hospitalization benefits per a menu of covered medications and services. Benefits are designed to provide coverage for those who are not eligible for IMSS. Enrollment is available to foreigners holding temporary or permanent resident's visa and the cost is on a sliding scale. There are no age restrictions and pre-existing conditions are covered. [*See Seguro Popular, Secretaría de Salud (SSA)*]

Medicare & Medicaid

Treatment, hospitalization or emergency care (or payment or reimbursement for these) is not available in Mexico through the United State government Medicare or Medicaid programs at this time. While you can collect Social Security benefits anywhere and you can enroll in Medicare while living in Mexico if you qualify, the only medical care that is covered by Medicare, with rare exception, is that given within the United States borders and specific territories.

The rare exceptions are as follows:

1. If you have Medicare supplements F or N, you are covered for emergency/urgent care up to a lifetime limit of $50,000, $250 deductible, and the incident must occur no longer than 60 days after leaving the USA. You will typically have to pay personally and file a claim with Medicare.
2. Medicare is accepted only in the fifty states of the USA and the District of Colombia, Puerto Rico, Guam, the U.S. Virgin Islands, American Samoa, and the Northern Mariana Islands. Medicare will cover you on cruise ships provided they are within six hours of a U.S. port and the onboard physician treated you and determined you required emergency hospitalization (however, expect to pay the bill yourself and to submit a claim for reimbursement).
3. The other rare exception would be if you had a medical emergency while traveling in the U.S.A. and the nearest hospital were in Canada or Mexico. In that case you may be reimbursed for those hospital expenses. The same would be true if you were traveling through Canada on your way to or returning from Alaska.

As a consequence, many expats from the US consider Medicare an option to be used only when absolutely necessary since the expense of travel and the inconvenience and isolation (being away from friends and family in Mexico) may create an additional hardship during what may already be a difficult time. In the case of an accident or serious illness, those relying on Medicare may require medical evacuation, a very expensive proposition ($30,000–70,000) without evacuation insurance. So while you still have hospitalization coverage in the US, getting there can be impossible under some circumstances. [*See Air Evacuation Insurance*]

Nevertheless, there are those who do travel back the United States for more expensive treatments or procedures, have Medicare foot the bill, and then return to Mexico to live happily in health again.

While it is a popular notion among expats, and there have even been some lobbying efforts and discussion in some government circles about allowing Medicare to pay benefits in Mexico—an idea supported by a RAND Corporation study—it is unlikely in the current environment.[26]

Other Government-Sponsored Insurance

For many Europeans, Canadians and Australians who are unaccustomed to paying providers directly for medical care (or buying their own insurance)—you should be aware that there are no reciprocal agreements with Mexico. You will be entirely responsible for providing payment for any medical care you receive, with or without private insurance. If you want insurance, you must purchase it privately.

Private Clinic Programs & Discount Medical Memberships

While availability will vary from location to location, and the specific benefits are designed by the clinics or medical groups involved, a private clinic program may offer exactly the kind of medical services you and your family are likely to need for routine visits, home visits, discounts or hospitalization at specific private hospitals, reduced prices on medical treatment, etc.

Please keep in mind that these programs do not typically provide comprehensive hospital benefits and it might be difficult to collect the benefits under some circumstances. Please investigate the terms carefully. However, for some expats, these programs are a welcome addition and they express satisfaction. While you will have to investigate local options, here is a representative example: Medica Vrim,[27] Medicall Home.[28]

Funding Elective Surgery

Most insurance plans do not cover cosmetic surgery or other "elective" surgeries or treatments such as liposuction, bariatric surgery nor in most cases, help with infertility treatments. However, for some people, correcting a physical flaw, reducing dangerous levels of obesity, having a baby or perhaps having another chance at health and long life by trying an elective treatment isn't just an option: it is essential to their happiness and well-being and in some cases, their survival.

If your personal resources aren't adequate to pay for the treatment you need, or your traditional sources of funding—like borrowing against savings or taking a larger mortgage—aren't available to you, there is a branch of the finance industry that will consider financing elective surgery. While we don't endorse any particular companies that provide this service, we are committed to laying out the options and this is certainly one option in the whole spectrum. For example, there are websites that promote funding for elective surgery and that may be an option for some. For others, tapping their already-established lines of credit may make more sense.

Air Evacuation Insurance

If you are ill or injured in a country other than your home country, getting home for medical treatment may be your preferred option. After all, that is where your friends, family and familiar medical services are. You may need to return in order to take advantage of your home-grown insurance, Medicare or Medicaid.

But getting back home may not be as easy as buying a ticket and getting on the plane. In order to fly you have to be healthy enough to go through customs, through security, through the gate, sit in a seat for hours and handle possible layovers. Airports offer a toxic mix of bad food, long distances to walk or awkward wheelchair assists. If you have an infectious disease, you should not fly and endanger others. If your immune system is weakened, you should avoid exposure to the public.

One wise solution is to purchase Air Evacuation Insurance that assures that if you are hospitalized you will be escorted by medical professionals in a private jet to a hospital in your home country. Some policies will take you to the hospital of your choice (that accepts you) and help make all the arrangements with the receiving hospital so that a room will be ready for you when you arrive. They will help streamline any customs process and monitor you to make sure your condition is stable while you are traveling.

Air evacuation involves more than just a private jet flight. Yes, they have planes with pilots and medical personnel on standby. But in order to offer bed-to-bed service—where you are taken from one hospital room via ambulance to the nearest airport, across international borders (where you may need to change transport), to your destination city to another ambulance and finally delivered to the hospital of your choice (if that's what the terms of your policy says, and that agrees to admit you)—there are lots of logistics involved. The air evacuation company's staff is involved with every step along the way, consulting with medical personnel at both ends, confirming that you are stable, and assisting with the complex logistics involved in international border crossings of this kind.

Although an individual can work directly with an air evacuation company, the costs are high ($30,000-70,000 USD). As a far more affordable option, most people receive this service by purchasing Air Evacuation Insurance and the insurance company contracts with the actual air evacuation provider. Make sure to ask about the accreditations of the provider an insurer is contracting with and review the specific terms of the coverage carefully. For example, most will require that you be hospitalized in Mexico before you are evacuated.

While Air Evacuation Insurance is not necessarily an option needed for expats who plan to receive all of their medical care in Mexico, there are those who prefer being treated in their hometown, or by the medical staff of a particular hospital in another country. If that describes you, then Air Evacuation Insurance is an option you may want to consider.

As you can imagine, being able to relax while you are moved safely from a bed in one country to a bed in another could be very welcome under what might already be trying circumstances.

Lifestyle & Care Needs During Retirement

An Overview

With nearly 60 million American adults currently age 60 or older, and the numbers of senior citizens growing daily, the aging of the US population is a vast and timely trend and will be for years to come.

Baby Boomers have now reached retirement age and the need for independent living, assisted living and other long-term care options has never been greater. However, high costs for building, staffing, and managing facilities in the US have limited developer investment and the typical facility is not affordable by the majority of middle-class would-be residents.

Mexico offers the promise of good-quality, affordable options.

Retiree Income

A more in-depth look at the numbers reveals why assisted living in the US is not affordable for many seniors. The mean income of 48% of retirees 65 years and over in the US is $22,862. And that represents all sources of income, not just Social Security (collected by 91.5% of those 65 and over) at a mean of $18,123 annually.

Of those collecting Social Security, half started collecting before they had originally planned, while only 5% retired later than originally planned. Almost four in 10 respondents (37%) who retired earlier than they had planned cite health-related reasons for doing so.

The Costs and Payment for Assisted Living

In the United States between 75–90% of the cost of assisted living is paid out of pocket. Medicare, the major source of medical coverage for retirees, typically contributes nothing for living costs including independent and assisted living. The Canadian Long Term Care Funding Center Inc. states that, depending on where retirees reside, the monthly cost of long-term care can range between $2,800 and $9,000. Residents pay 70% of their after-tax income for a full package of services. Individuals with high income spend up to a maximum amount based on actual cost.

MetLife's Mature Market Institute puts the average rate for a stay at an assisted-living facility in the US at $3550 a month in 2012, up from $3477 in 2011. (No doubt it is higher today) With the mean retiree income at $22,862 annually, and the average cost of assisted living at $42,600 annually, there is obviously a huge "affordability" gap.

Nursing home care typically runs higher, up to $9750 per month. The national average daily rate for a private room in a nursing home is $248, while a semi-private room is $222 (up from $239 and $214 respectively in 2011).

Even the cost for in-home care support is prohibitive for many in the US. The national average hourly rate for home-health aides is $21, while the average hourly rate for a homemaker is $20 in 2012 was.

For some, Mexico can fill the gap. As of the publication of this edition of *The English Speaker's Guide to Medical Care in Mexico*, the exchange rate is over 20 Mexican pesos to a single US dollar. This offers those with incomes in dollars an amazing advantage, although that will vary over time and the advantage is likely to be diminished slightly by inflation as prices increase. Nevertheless, there is no doubt that your US or Canadian income will go much further in Mexico; perhaps twice as far for many expenditures.

Defining Independent & Assisted Living

The goal of both independent and assisted living facilities is to offer a healthy lifestyle and needed safety and care for seniors. The type of care required for retirees ranges from almost no specialized care, to total dependency and full-time nursing care.

The categories that most concern us here, by degree of need, are "independent living" where housekeeping help is standard and a supplemental menu of available services can be utilized on an "as needed" basis, and "assisted living" where more extensive care is needed and an entire menu of services are typically included for a monthly fee. You will need to shop for the kind of lifestyle you are seeking. [*See Appendix J: Retirement Communities, Assisted Living & Nursing Care*]

Independent Living & Retirement Communities

For a growing number of people, there is a period of time between retirement and the end of life when we are healthy and prefer to live as independently as possible. If we have been financially careful or lucky, we have the means to live a relatively luxurious life in Mexico. Even if you have not amassed significant financial resources, as long as you have a regular income based on something other than working in the Mexican economy, US Social Security for example, you can probably find a comfortable way of living in Mexico. But for those who can afford the amenities, there are whole retirement communities that are built around a lifestyle that offers a menu of everything from a place to moor your yacht to hotel-like concierge services.

If you fall into this category, you are what marketers refer to as an "active adult." While you could easily purchase or rent a stand-alone home, the the idea of living in a community of people you share much in common with has its appeal. So, whether your sport is golf or tennis, fishing or biking, or if you prefer trips to galleries and to view colonial architecture, you can find a planned retirement community to suit your taste, although they may be beyond your means.

Assisted Living & Nursing Home Care

As we age, our need for medical and other types of care inevitably increases whether we live on our own or not. Our eyesight and our joints weaken and for some of us, living alone is no longer a suitable option.

In traditional cultures like Mexico's, this is not a problem. There is seldom a question about what will happen. The elderly live with their children or other close relatives until the end of life, just as their children lived with them typically until marriage. Most elderly people are loved and respected. And, in a culture where there are relatively fewer elderly people (30% of the population is 14 or under and the median age is 26) it is not unusual for children, teens and young adults to be sensitive to the needs of the elderly around them and offer a helping hand on the street.

In the US and many other western countries, living with one's children is not always seen as a reasonable option for aging parents. Attitudes about independence are different and elderly parents are reluctant to become a logistical or financial "burden" on their children. The need for living options has driven a whole industry: to provide assisted living and nursing home care for the elderly.

In the United States, the quality of care ranges from the very good to the frighteningly bad. The cost of providing this kind of care is enormous: $1800 to $5000 per month and 75–90% of the cost is paid out of pocket in the US where Medicare contributes nothing to assisted living cost. MetLife's Mature Market Institute puts the average rate for an assisted-living facility in the U.S. at $3,031 a month. (Nursing home care typically runs higher, up to $9000 per month.)

Furthermore, in the US culture, caring for elderly people is considered a low-status job. So the elderly living on fixed incomes without savings or assets are often forced to live in environments where they are little more than warehoused and where the care is marginal or worse. It can be a depressing way to end one's life.

Assisted living and nursing home care is a relatively new concept in Mexico. After all, this is a culture where the vast majority of elderly people live with family members. Those facilities that existed in the past were traditionally run as charities. However, the business and healthcare communities of both Mexico and the United States have begun to invest in care facilities in Mexico that are planned to serve the elderly from other parts of the world with the expectation of increasing demand. The demographics support their optimism.

In the US, over 8,000 adults per day turn age 60. Most of them will have to work beyond traditional retirement age in order to support themselves and even then, a comfortable future is not assured. Increasingly life in Mexico becomes a solution for the elderly and their families since the cost of assisted living is 30-50% of what equivalent care might be in one's home country.

An estimated 10 to 15 million people will be seeking retirement or care in Mexico by 2025, a trend that is encouraged by the Mexican government. For some, it will be possible to live at home longer because household help is affordable. Furthermore, since the salaries for nurses are low (approximately $550 per month), full- or part-time in-home nursing care is also an option for many.

While assisted-living care in Mexico may be less expensive, it is not monitored nor licensed and not all facilities offer quality care. There are currently no screening agencies evaluating and rating facilities, and finding one that might be suitable for you or a family member is strictly an ad hoc affair.

Typical Features of Assisted Living

HelpGuide.org indicates that the typical features of assisted living facilities are as follows:

- Three meals per day in common area which serves as dining room
- Help with eating meals, bathing and dressing, going to the bathroom, as well as walking.
- Housekeeping activities;
- Transportation;
- Access to health care;
- Security throughout the day – 24-hour security;
- Call systems for emergency in each living area;
- Wellness programs including regular exercise;
- Management of medication;
- Washing and ironing clothes;
- Activities for recreation and to enable socialization;
- Employees to help with both scheduled and unscheduled activities

This list does not guarantee these services will be provided, but rather gives you a kind of checklist that can guide your pursuit and help you compare the list of standard services provided between assisted living facilities.

The Pluses and Minuses

It is common for assisted care facilities in Mexico to also offer Internet service, libraries, video games, cable or satellite television in English and other electronic and telecommunications amenities. Some offer luxury features such as swimming pools, patios, exercise-machine-equipped gyms, putting greens, landscaped walkways and bike paths. The presence of medical staff on a 24-hour basis is an option for larger assisted living facilities.

You will need to interview representatives of each facility to discover what the costs are, what exactly is included in that cost and how financial and transportation arrangements are made. Keep a list of questions handy and voice any concerns you may have. Ask to review a written copy of any agreement in English, or have it translated before signing. We highly recommend that you visit the top two or three facilities before making a choice.

There are particular challenges if you are seeking care for a family member who will live far away from you. Even when you have done your best to find a workable solution, things don't always work out the way you planned in Mexico. New arrivals may find that the adjustment to living in a new country and unfamiliar surroundings is insurmountable leading to depression. A much-loved staff member leaves his or her job, the facility moves across the road and no longer has beach access, your elderly mother requires hospitalization: These are the normal complexities of life in Mexico and not necessarily failure on anyone's part.

If you are interested in working with a consultant who will help you by interviewing you about your needs, researching the appropriate options and then reviewing them with you, please contact the author.[29]

End-of-Life Issues

Making Your Intentions Known

There are many people who do not wish for their lives to be prolonged by artificial means if the quality of their lives would be minimal. For example, they don't want to be sustained in a vegetative state. Citizens from the US, Canada and the UK are familiar with "Do Not Resuscitate" orders or "Living Wills" and many have completed them in conjunction to hospitalization (although you often have to ask for the papers specifically).

At the time of the writing of the first edition of this book there were few rights for patients once they entered a hospital in Mexico. You might be guaranteed treatment, but once started, it could not be stopped by the patient. Now, however, there is a new national law that allows the patient to direct their own terminal care using an advance healthcare directive expressed in a letter.

The new law, known as *Reforma 39: Ley General de Salud,* was enacted by the Mexican Congress and signed into law by the then president Felipe Calderón in 2009 to provide you with the legal basis for expressing your wishes regarding palliative care (pain relief and comfort care) even if you are not capable of making informed decisions. (The law allows you to designate someone to make medical decisions for you if you are not able.) The law applies to those who are terminally ill and not expected to survive over six months.

The actual law can be found in an appendix at the end of this book [*See Appendix K: Mexico's Palliative Care* Law], or it can be downloaded from a government website in Spanish.[30] This might be needed if you find that your local caregivers are unfamiliar with the law. Frankly, most are not. In fact, many of them will even tell you about an older law that only applied in Mexico City and required the expensive services of a Notary. Respect that this is a relatively new law and it is likely that not everyone will be aware of it. You may be the one to provide the education, but you will need a copy of the actual law to back up your claims. I recommend that you attach a copy of the law in Spanish to any letter of direction you sign. [*See Preparing an End-of-Life Care Document*]

We Must End Suffering

Despite the national law intended to help and empower all Mexicans to have access to palliative care at the end of life, many still suffer with horrific levels of pain before death. Genuine end-of-life palliative care often calls for the administration of controlled substances such as morphine to control pain.[31] Finding a doctor able and willing to prescribe pain medications in Mexico can be challenging in the face of ignorance about the law of the land and the fact that not all doctors can prescribe controlled substances. Finding a pharmacy willing and able to dispense morphine or other palliative drugs is another current barrier to providing proper end-of-life care. [*See Which Type of Pharmacy Do You Need?*]

While we cannot always prolong life, we can almost always help those we love end their days in peace and comfort if we are able to engage the help of knowledgeable doctors and pharmacists. One way to help now—to actually change the current culture of Mexico before you or your loved one needs palliative care—is is to let others know about the law. Tell your friends and family. Tell your doctors. Give them a copy of the actual law. Complete your own advance healthcare directive letter and let your doctors and family know about it. If you are in assisted living, please have a copy of your directive placed in your file.

Highlights of the Law

Although the law and the documents used to convey your wishes are in Spanish (and you should complete the Spanish version of the documents), here is a link to a side-by-side Spanish/English Google translation of Title 8 (the section of the law that applies) prepared by the late beloved expert on Mexico, Rolly Brooks.[32] There are four chapters that apply and here are some of the highlights. (It is highly recommended that you read the entire law.)

Chapter I

Establishes the purpose of the law and provides definitions of several terms used in the law. Among these provisions are:

Palliative Care: Is the total active care of those illnesses that cannot be cured. The goal is the control of pain and other symptoms, and psychological care, social and spiritual. (Chapter I, Article 166, Bis 1, III.)

Pain management: All those measures provided by health professionals, designed to reduce physical and emotional suffering of a terminal illness product, designed to improve the quality of life. (Chapter I, Article 166, Bis 1, IX)

Chapter II

Establishes the rights of terminally ill patients. Among these provisions are:

To voluntarily leave the health institution where they are hospitalized. (Chapter II, Art. 166, Bis 3, III).

To receive clear, timely and sufficient information on the conditions and effects of their disease and types of treatments which can be chosen. (Chapter II, Art. 166, Bis 3, V)

To ask the doctor to administer medication to mitigate the pain; resign or leave at any time, refuse to receive or continue treatment considered extraordinary; elect to receive hospice care in a private home (Chapter II, Art 166, Bis 1, VII - IX)

A patient in a terminal situation while still able to make informed decisions, has the right to order the session of curative medical treatments and to change to a palliative treatment focused exclusively on the reduction of pain in the form and terms provided in this law. (Chapter II, Art. 166, Bis 5/6).

The law allows patients to designate a person authorized to make medical decisions for them if they are unable to make their own informed decisions. (Chapter II, Art. 166, Bis 3, X); and for patients to express their wishes for end of life care in a written health care directive. (Chapter II, Art. 166, Bis 4).

Relatives of terminally ill patients have the obligation to respect decisions the patient voluntarily takes in terms of this law. (Chapter II, Art. 166, Bis 10).

In cases of medical emergency and there is inability of the patient in a situation terminal to consent, in the absence of relatives, legal representative, guardian or person trust, the decision to implement a medical procedure or surgical treatment necessary will be made by the specialist and/or by the Bioethics Committee of the institution. (Chapter II, Art. 166, Bis 11)

Chapter III

Powers and Duties of Health Facility. Among these provisions are:

Provide palliative care for the type and extent of disease, from time of diagnosis of terminal illness until the last moment; create specialized areas to care for terminally ill patients; and provide training and updating of human resources in the field of palliative care and care for terminally ill patients. (Chapter III, Art 166, Bis 12, IV - VI)

Chapter IV

Rights, powers and duties of medical and health workers. Among these provisions are:

Provide all required information to patient that the doctor feels necessary for the patient to make a free and informed decision about treatment and care. (Chapter IV, Art 166, Bis 15, I)

Respect the decision of terminally ill patients in curative treatment and palliative care, once the doctor has explained in simple terms the consequences of the patient's decision. (Chapter IV, Art 166, Bis 15, V)

Attending physicians may provide palliative drugs to a patient in terminal situation, even when doing so causes a lose of alertness or shortens the life of the patient, provided that these drugs provide palliative care with the aim of alleviating the patient's pain. (Chapter IV, Art. 166, Bis 16). There are strict probations against using these drugs for euthanasia. (Chapter IV, Art 166, Bis 16)

Preparing an End-of-Life Care Document

It is important that you prepare a healthcare directive letter to give medical staff, family members and others that outlines exactly the care you wish to receive (or not receive) at the end your life. The law allows you to prepare the document yourself. There is no requirement that you use a lawyer to prepare it. However, your end-of-life care document *must* be in Spanish since Spanish is the official language of Mexico. So, you may need help preparing it.

Here is what you need to do:

Read the law so that you understand what provisions you really wish to invoke. Once you have put your intentions in writing and given them to medical professionals, it may cause great confusion and disruption to attempt to change your directions.

Before designating someone who will be authorized to make medical decisions for you, discuss your wishes to be sure the person actually understands what you are asking them to do and is willing to act faithfully on your behalf. Provide a copy of your health care directive and the law.

Your healthcare directive should clearly state what care you want or don't want. It must be based on what is in the law. It would be wise to include references to the paragraph in the law that supports your directive, as you will find in the sample directive. (A sample directive letter in both English and Spanish is at the end of this book.) [*See Appendix L: Sample Health Care Directive Letter*]

If you have a question about exactly what medical directives to include or how to word the directives, discuss it with your doctor. Take a copy of the law with you to be sure the doctors and other medical staff understand its requirements.[33]

Sign and date the letter in the presence of two witnesses. Then the witnesses will also sign it.

Give a copy to your primary care doctor along with a copy of the law in Spanish. When you are hospitalized, provide a copy to the medical staff, again with a copy of the law in Spanish. If you are in assisted living, give the administration a copy to put in your file.

Hospice Care

Hospice care is designed to give supportive assistance to people in the final phases of a terminal illness and focus on comfort and quality of life, rather than cure. The hospice philosophy is to help terminally or seriously ill patients by treating pain and symptoms, and attending to their emotional and spiritual needs. The goal is to enable patients to be comfortable and free of pain, so that they live each day as fully as possible.

Another goal of hospice care is to give "respite" (relief) for primary care givers (typically a spouse, friend or family member) so that they can have time off to attend to their personal needs. As such, hospice care can be delivered by medical professionals, family and friends, church members, nurses, housekeepers and other care givers. Hospice care is typically given at the very end of life and may utilize a team approach.

While any willing doctor can provide hospice medical care, and it is common in Mexico for friends and family to provide hospice-like support for each other, there are also a growing number of organizations in Mexico that provide or arrange hospice care as well.

As with many new medical trends, you are more likely to access a hospice care organization in a city, for example, there are many in Mexico City, but the number is growing all the time and your doctor, church or local hospital may be able to help connect you with local hospice care. There are also organizations online that may be able to help.[34]

Upon Your Death in Mexico

If you are living in Mexico, it is an excellent idea to have a will that specifies what you would like to be done with your body if you should die in Mexico (especially addressing if it will be returned to your homeland) and the distribution of your assets in Mexico. You should do this even if you have a will that outlines the same things in your home country so that your executor does not have to have your English will translated and filed in Mexico after your death.

Although any will would be honored, the complexities can be considerably reduced by having a Mexican will already prepared. Wills are prepared and filed by Notaries in Mexico, not lawyers. You can typically get a good referral through social networking although in small towns there may only be one or two options.

All deaths, births and marriages in Mexico must be registered with the Mexican authorities at the *Registro Civil*.

If the body is to travel, those arrangements should be made by a funeral home in Mexico. They are authorized by law to make the arrangements and prepare the paperwork and they can work with funeral homes in other countries to speed the process. The funeral home in the US should also be notified in order to speed things on the other side of the border.

If one dies without clear instructions or family members in Mexico, their home country's Embassy will do whatever they can to find family and notify them of the death, but clearly this is hardly ideal.

Foreign Medical Program for Disabled US Veterans

If you are a disabled United States veteran, it is possible for you to enjoy the benefits of living or traveling abroad, while at the same time taking advantage of the medical care you are entitled to from the United States Department of Veteran's Affairs. You can live anywhere you want with a few exceptions: Cuba, and Iraq (or Canada and the Philippines where there are other programs in place). There is no reason to stay in the US unless you want to. You are free to travel or live where you wish.

Why Isn't This Benefit Better Known?

When we discovered that there was a Foreign Medical Program for disabled US Veterans, we found this information both surprising and interesting. For one thing, there just didn't seem to be a lot of information about it. For another, it seemed that this knowledge might really open up some opportunities to improve the lifestyle of many disabled veterans.

But why isn't information about benefit better known? It would take an expert on Veteran's affairs to answer that question, but it could be that by talking about the fact that the government will pay for your medical care wherever in the world you want to live they risk looking like they are encouraging people to leave the country. Or worse: they might be falsely accused of tying to dump veterans on other healthcare systems. It is easy to see how they might be criticized for that. But, we think people should be made aware of what's available so they can decide what's best for themselves.

Why Consider Living Outside the USA?

There are a lot of reasons people might choose to live outside of the United States. For some people, it might be simply to return to your families' country of origin or homeland. For others, it might be to marry or to join children in another land. But for many others it because living outside of the US could provide a higher standard of living and better-quality care.

Even with full benefits, including medical care, the cost of living in the United States may be prohibitively high. Options for in-home care are limited and housing may be prohibitively expensive. However, if you are no longer tethered to the US by your need for medical care, you may experience a better quality of care, and a better quality of life, outside of the US.

A Better Quality of Life May Be Possible

Of course, what is "better" is subjective and living in a foreign country isn't for everyone. But for some moving to another country could offer a much needed improvement. For example, living in Mexico could offer a disabled veteran all of the normal veteran benefits (including medical care) plus enough in the monthly budget for good quality housing, part- or full-time household help (including cooking), in-home medical assistance, physician house calls, etc. Add to this the possibility of a nearby beach or swimming pool, a culture that offers respect to veterans and the elderly and whose citizens consider providing personal care honorable work. With direct flights between many major cities in the US and Mexico, visits to and from friends and family are realistic as well.

Before you pick up and leave, you are going to want to research the possibilities carefully and even visit the most likely places more than once before making your move. You need to discover the local circumstances by actually exploring the environment and doing a lot of online research. We also recommend that you engage in social networking and begin to make friends in Mexico today. [*See Expat Groups for Medical Referrals & Social Networking*]

What Will You Need?

For example, consider: will it be possible to bring your car or purchase one with modifications if you need them? What about mobility? Are residential neighborhoods accessible to those in a wheelchair or with other physical challenges getting around? [*See There are Mobility Issues*] What about accessibility of stores and services like hospitals and doctor's offices? Can you easily purchase the medicines and equipment you need?

To continue with the example of Mexico, the idea of accessibility is relatively new there. Although those with disabilities are given full legal rights, getting around on cobbled streets that lack curb cuts might be a factor in many locations. If you use a wheelchair or have difficulty walking, you would want to consider where you relocated carefully. For example, good places in Mexico might be Querétaro, a modern city with a focus on the international business community and the site of a lot of newer, more accessible construction or Lake Chapala where there is a large community of expats including US veterans who may be able to provide a built-in social network for support.

Housing is also a consideration. Can you buy a house or will you rent? Do you need modifications? If so, how will those be arranged?

Obviously, each person has to make their own evaluation based on their own situation, but nearly 20,000 disabled veterans are currently living outside the US, many of them in Mexico, so clearly there are many who felt that ex-patriot-living offered a viable option.

Here's Where to Apply

If you have been verified as disabled by the Veteran's Administration you should quality for the Foreign Medical Program benefits. Ask about the Foreign Medical Program (FMP) at the Department of Veterans Affairs.

If You Are Moving to Mexico

For readers who are considering Mexico as your new residence, whether because of job opportunities, retirement or family, there are a number of health-related factors that should weigh in your decision about where to live. This is the list of what may be the most important. Many of these are addressed elsewhere in this book.

Health Considerations in Choosing a Location in Mexico

- Availability of Hospitals [*See Appendix A: The English Speakers Guide to Doctors & Hospitals in Mexico*]
- Doctors & Specialists —This is especially important if you are being treated by a specialist for a chronic health condition. Medical specialist in Mexico will not be found in every community where expats congregate. [*See Appendix C: Medical Specialties & Medical Boards*]
- Seasonal Temperature & Humidity — The Winter weather at the beach may be ideal, but high summer temperatures could be a different story and air-conditioning may be essential. Some high altitude cities and towns have warm, sunny days, but the nights are cold and there is no central heating.
- Altitude — This could be important if you have asthma, emphysema or other breathing difficulties [*See Problems with Altitude*]
- Availability of Necessary Pharmaceuticals — [*See Finding Your Medicine in Mexico*]
- Social Isolation— Not having friends and family nearby can adversely affect your health. There are ways to compensate, but it doesn't happen magically. [*See Problems with Altitude*]
- Emergency Response [*See Uncertain Emergency Response*]
- Mobility [*See There are Mobility Issues*]

Medical Tourism

Medical tourism is a booming worldwide industry that is driven by the need for affordable quality care or treatments that are not available in the United States, Canada or the United Kingdom. Many people in these countries have been driven out of their local markets by high costs, insurance exclusions, their desire for non-approved treatments or long waiting times for treatments doled out by government programs.

Americans and Canadians often have very different motivations for traveling to Mexico for medical treatment.

Most Americans seek medical options in Mexico for economic reasons. Typically, the cost of the procedure they need or want is beyond their means in the US. Most often this is because they are uninsured, under-insured (deductibles and co-pays would leave them broke) or the procedure they are seeking is not covered at all. They may not even be offered the best solution because of the expense involved. [*See Los Algodones and Dental Implants*] Whatever their situation, it boils down to economics.

For Canadians it is a different matter. The more important consideration is time rather than money. While most healthcare costs for necessary treatment are actually paid by the various provincial governments, the amount of "wait time" can be considerable: months, not days.

The amount of time you must wait varies based on where you live and the service or procedure you need. Needless to say, when you are the one confined to a wheelchair awaiting hip-replacement surgery for example, there may be a sense that you are losing precious time, a chunk of your life you will never get back. Pain and disability are poor trade-offs for the economic benefit of government provided care.

Furthermore, there may be multiple "wait times" for those procedures in high demand: a wait of weeks to see a specialist, another lengthy wait for diagnostic tests, another wait of months, perhaps as much as year or more from start to finish for an essential surgery, and so on.

Canadians understandably obsess about waiting. In fact, there is a 98-page document entitled "Waiting Your Turn" that gives approximate wait times to see a specialist or to schedule a procedure based on where one lives. A recent survey of Canadian doctors by the Fraser Institute reveals that, "wait times in Canada are longer than what physicians consider to be clinically reasonable," so even doctors feel the wait times are detrimental for their patients.

Waiting is the reason many Canadians who have the resources to pay for the treatment they need simply don't wait. In fact, approximately 40% of the visitors who come to Mexico for medical care are Canadians who have decided that life is too short to be disabled by the lack of a needed surgery. Why suffer pain and physical limitation when excellent, affordable care—including the specialists, diagnostics and surgery—is available immediately in Mexico? Why wait if you don't have to?

Surprisingly, people often find that the kindness and care are better than they could expect to find in their own country and the medical standards are on a par with what they have available at home. Couple this with quick accessibility, friendly staff and helpful extras like room and board for a family member or an escort to and from the airport and is it any wonder that offshore options are increasingly inviting? So, many people who might not have received treatment at all—anything from a hip replacement to fertility treatments—have been successfully and affordably treated and have spread the word and thus the number of people being served increases all the time.

Today there are dozens of affordable medical procedures that are available in Mexico. These include organ transplants including kidney, liver, and stem cell transplants, heart surgery, fertility treatment, laparoscopic surgery, weight-loss procedures for obesity treatment such as bariatrics, cosmetic procedures including breast reduction and augmentation, rhinoplasty (nose surgery), liposuction and face lifts, orthopedic surgeries including knee, hip and other joint replacements, a wide variety of dental procedures including dental implants and eye surgeries, including cornea transplants and lasik eye surgery.

In addition to all the standard treatments, many medical tourists come to Mexico for alternative medical therapies performed by licensed doctors that are not approved or available in their home countries. [*See Alternative Therapies in Mexico*]

Cost Savings & More

Mexico is one of the countries with an extensive list of medical providers for the medical tourist, and because of the geographical proximity to the United States it is a preferred destination. In fact, many treatment centers are in border cities to make transportation faster and less expensive.

While there are many types of treatment offered in Mexico that are of interest to the medical tourist, and this book presents information about the most popular treatments, particularly those high-cost treatments that offer a clear price advantage, in truth nearly any treatment you might want will be available in Mexico, most for 20-50% of the cost the equivalent treatment would be in your home country. One way of keeping costs even lower may be to steer away from those clinics that specifically target the medical tourist and seek treatment in the institutions where Mexicans themselves typically receive treatment.

We can only approximate cost comparison data for common medical procedures in the US and Mexico because of the regional differences and frequent changes in exchange rates. While every situation is different, and these figures are intended to be representative, the savings is obvious. [*See Appendix M: Cost Comparisons, USA & Mexico*]

If you are pursuing other types of care, including joint replacement, obesity treatment or cosmetic surgery, we recommend seeking a referral from the boards that provide certification in the specialty you need. [*See Medical Board Certification & Medical Specialties*] You also might consider using a reputable international referral organization such as MedtoGo.[35]

Questions Medical Tourists to Mexico Need to Ask

People from the United States and Canada have been traveling south to Mexico for medical treatment for decades. This includes people in the border regions who simply find care on "*el otro lado*" convenient and familiar, especially for those who have roots in Mexico, and also to those needing major surgeries such as an organ transplant or hip replacement and find that care in their home country is not affordable or will be delayed for months.

While there are many facilities that crow about the quality of their medical care and how modern their facilities are, it can be difficult to evaluate them objectively. Sometimes potential "medical tourists" (people traveling for medical care) don't even know what to ask to help them decide where to go for treatment. While this is not necessarily a complete list—you will have questions that are specific to your unique needs—it should help you in your quest.

Questions you need to ask:

- How far you are able to travel in comfort? (air travel over long distances is not appropriate for all medical tourists)
- What kinds of certification and accreditation does the facility have?
- What are the areas of specialization of the hospital you are considering?
- Who are the doctors who would be treating you and what training have they had?
- Do the doctors and staff speak your native language?
- How often has the surgical team performed the procedure you are seeking?
- What is their success rate with that procedure?
- Are the doctors board-certified in the specialty you require?
- What recommendations or testimonials can be provided related to your specific medical needs?
- Are there former patients you can speak to or correspond with?
- What is the package of accommodations and services you are being offered?
- Can the hospital or clinic provide any special dietary or mobility needs you have?
- What is the price, and what is specifically included in that price?
- Will there be any additional charges?
- What provisions have been made for after-surgery care and follow up treatment?
- What kind of relationship are you able to build with the facilitator or provider? Are you comfortable with them?

Combining Surgery with an Amazing Vacation

When I first learned about medical tourism many years ago, I was impressed that good quality, affordable medical care was available to nearly everyone if they were willing to travel. But the "tourism" part didn't register with me as being very important. However, now I've had an opportunity to visit Los Cabos and meet many of the medical professionals in the area, I have a whole new point of view: I think it is actually worth planning a vacation around a medical or dental procedure. It might even be one of the best vacations of your life.

The Los Cabos region is on the southern-most tip of Baja California Sur. It's warm and sunny there nearly all-year with temperatures typically in the 80's (cooler at night), and with balmy sea breezes. In fact, it rains so seldom that rain tends to be a cause for celebration and you'd want to stop to appreciate the rare phenomena of a desert landscape in bloom.

The area known as Los Cabos is composed of two main towns—Cabo San Lucas and San Jose del Cab—each with its own unique character, and the corridor between them is dotted with quality hotels and resorts. Both towns are served by an international airport with regular flights from many major cities in the U.S. and Canada. So, it's easy to get there and there are plenty of places to stay. Although Los Cabos is one of the more upscale destinations in Mexico, working with a local medical facilitator will help you access good rates on local accommodations and other services. [*See About Medical Facilitation*]

Los Cabos is also an ideal place to convalesce following medical treatment. In addition to a choice of accommodations including charming boutique hotels and high quality resorts–all of which offer outstanding personal service–you will also have access to delicious and nutritious fresh foods to aid your recovery, including fruits and vegetables, fresh juices, seafood, and a variety of regional and international cuisine.

The area has become a magnet for top medical professionals, some of whom live and work in Los Cabos full-time, others who practice in both Mexico City and Los Cabos making weekly flights between the two. Most doctors and surgeons work with either Amerimed, a modern private hospital that has served the area for years, or American British Cowdray hospital, a new state-of-the-art facility operated by the ABC chain of hospitals.

About Medical Facilitation

A medical facilitator is an individual that assists a patient in making the complex medical, transportation and living arrangements required to set up medical treatment in a foreign country. Among the advantages of working with a medical facilitator is the day-to-day relationship they form with the local practitioners and their staff. Facilitators can also help with aspects of your travel and treatment, for example, booking your air transport and accommodations, making your medical appointments, receiving you at the airport, and providing local transportation.

You may be able to travel to Mexico, receive treatment from a top medical professional, stay in a lovely hotel and recover in comfort amidst beautiful surroundings for a week while eating tasty, nutritious fresh food and having all the arrangements made for you–and still pay less than you'd pay for the medical treatment alone in the U.S. or Canada. A medical facilitator can make it all happen smoothly.

If you have the budget and you'd like to enjoy a relaxing vacation in the sun while getting excellent medical treatment, we recommend considering working with a facilitator with Cabo Health Travel.[36] This organization provides trustworthy referrals and many services for people looking for medical services for various orthopedic, cardiac and cosmetic surgeries and other standard procedures.

The Most Critical Need for Medical Tourists

I recently did some research to discover which health issues people consulted Google for to find medical information. I was expecting a long list of diseases and conditions and, of course, that's what I got. In fact, I found there were 323 keywords related to common health issues that had significant numbers of monthly searches globally.

What I wasn't expecting was how one particular category of medical search was so disproportionally large. I was surprised by both the numbers of people searching for information, and what exactly they were looking for. I must admit that I had no idea this health issue was so pervasive, and while the number of searches aren't the same as the number of people who have a disease, the search numbers can give some insight. Can you guess what the disease is?

If you answered practically anything related to heart health, you'd be right. The numbers simply floored me.

Here are some examples: "cardiology" was searched for 1,500,000 times a month globally and 823,000 times a month just in the United States. Additionally, "cardiologist" was searched for 1,000,000 times a month globally and 550,000 times a month in the United States.

Now, you might search for a cardiologist just to find someone to perform a routine EKG exam. But what about the 301,000 people (201,000 in the United States) who search for information on "bypass surgery" every month? I don't think those were all kids working on their homework. In fact, it doesn't take a leap of imagination to realize that literally hundreds of thousands of people are looking on Google for potentially life-saving information because they have just received a heart-related diagnosis. (WebMed.com states that 500,000 bypass surgeries are performed in the US every year.)

The information they will find about procedure costs won't be encouraging. For example, the cost of a heart bypass surgery in the United States is typically between $80,000 and $250,000—and that doesn't include the doctor's fees, or many of the necessary extras, such as pharmaceuticals. Fortunately, for many people much of the cost is likely to be covered with insurance. However, even for those with insurance, a 20% out-of-pocket co-payment on $250,000 hospital bill ($50,000) might place this potentially life-saving surgery out of reach, and for those without insurance…

Fortunately, it isn't hopeless. The international community has stepped-in to fill the void with affordable heart surgeries. Counties like India and Mexico are often able to perform the same procedures in Joint Commission accredited hospitals with board-certified surgical teams for a fraction of what it costs in the US. The quality of care is comparable (some would argue it is even better for the medical tourist), and for those who can't currently consider a necessary surgery because of the out-of-pocket costs, these options may be literally life-saving.

The very best heart-health treatment is prevention. Heart disease prevention and risk reduction is possible by living a healthy lifestyle; key advice includes:

- If needed, achieve medical control of diabetes, high blood pressure, and cholesterol
- Never smoke, or stop smoking cigarettes
- Eat a nutritious diet (many vegetables and fruits; less fats, sugars, and meats)
- Get at least 30 minutes of exercise almost every day
- Avoid alcohol, or consume no more than 1 drink per day for women and no more than 2 drinks per day for men

Transplantation of Organs, Tissues & Cells

There are many medical institutions in Mexico that are qualified to perform organ transplants including kidney, liver, heart and lung organ transplants as well as bone marrow, cornea, etc. According to the *Secretariá de Salud* (Secretary of Health) there are currently hundreds of hospitals licensed to perform transplants.

While thousands of transplants have been performed, the most common being kidney transplants, there has been historical shortage of donors in Mexico—a deficit of over 100,000. While efforts to generate awareness of the need for donors has increased and the laws were changed in 2000 to encourage donation, the waiting list for organs still far outpaces availability. For example, while 16 new patients with renal insufficiency are added to the list each day, only two or three patients receive a kidney. Thus it is unlikely that organs will be available for foreigners.

However, many types of organ transplants can be done with living donors—typically close family members—and with great success. While the cost of such transplants can be astronomically high in the United States, Canada or the UK, they will be significantly less expensive in Mexico. Thus, hospitals that are authorized to perform these surgeries may be of interest to the medical tourist.

Organ transplants in Mexico are overseen by the *Centro Nacional de Trasplantes* (CENATRA), part of the *Secretaría de Salud*.[37] While there maybe little to no opportunity to find suitable donor within the Mexican health system, CENATRA will be able to provide current information on hospitals that are approved to perform surgical transplants.

The following are private and university hospitals from the CENATRA list that are licensed to perform transplants by the listed by state and city (or *delegacion* in the case of Distrito Federal). While these only represent two categories of the hospitals that are approved to perform transplants, they are the ones that are typically available to medical tourists. The others are either part of the IMSS, ISSSTE or Pemex systems. Although foreigners with a resident's visa can enroll in IMSS or *Seguro Popular*, surgery of this kind is strictly controlled through internal referral.

If you are in need of an organ transplant, you most probably do not need fundamental information. Your path through the medical system has probably included a great deal more data about your medical options (or lack of them)—more than you ever wanted to know. What you may not be aware of is that knowledge about transplants goes back to the Aztec period in Mexico, a country that may be able to provide the healing surgery you need.

You will find many skilled surgical teams in Mexico who can help you if a living organ donor is available. Mexico can provide near immediate surgery and care for a fraction of what it would cost in the United States, Canada or the United Kingdom.

So, while no one can promise you the organ you may need, we are able to provide you with a list of those private hospitals in Mexico that are permitted by health authorities to provide transplants along with the specific procedures they are authorized to preform here: [*See Appendix F: Private Hospitals by State & City*]

Weight Loss (Bariatric) Surgery

Mexico was in the news recently when the United Nations Food and Agricultural Organization released a report showing Mexico's adult obesity rate had overtaken the United States adult obesity rate by one percentage point. While that one-point lead is well within the margins of error for data collection and reporting, the statistic will no less be ringing some bells on desks at the Mexican health ministry.

Although obesity is often associated with poor nutrition and inactive lifestyles, the issue is more complex than this and many factors including genetics, hormones, and stress are all believed to play a role in what has become one of the most pressing health issues of our age. The costs of obesity are well documented: an increased risk for heart disease, stroke, and diabetes to name a few.

For all of the health risks involved in being obese, there has traditionally been little support for those seeking to resolve the problem. For example, most employee health benefits do not include nutritional counseling or exercise programs and insurance policies often exclude any coverage for procedures designed to help control weight. The prevailing attitude has often been: "No one put a gun to your head and made you eat." As a result, medical treatment often comes late when more serious conditions arise.

As we've learned more about obesity, for example, that there isn't always a direct relationship between calorie intake and weight gain, attitudes are slowly changing. The American Medical Association recently announced that they are now considering obesity a disease. This opens the way for more research, insurance coverage and earlier medical intervention, but these sea-changes take time.

Meanwhile, Mexico is able to offer immediate solutions for many who seek relief from the effects of obesity. The country is the home of numerous surgeons, medical practices, hospitals and clinics that specialize in the most common weight control (Bariatric) procedures: lap band, gastric bypass, and gastric sleeve surgeries.

While the intention here is not to recommend specific surgeries, or specific medical practices, for thousands of obese people Mexico has offered amazing, life altering results. Like so many high-cost procedures that may be unaffordable in the US, or delayed in Canada, Mexico can offer immediate help at affordable prices in clean, modern medical facilities where well-trained medical staff and skilled surgical teams attend patients. While not every expectation is met, nor every procedure goes as planned—as is true anywhere weight-loss surgeries are performed—it is fascinating to hear what the patients themselves have to say about their weight-loss surgery experiences in Mexico.[38]

Breast Surgery

In theory at least, pretty much everyone likes breasts. Be they itty-bitty or mega-grande, from infancy through adulthood, breasts are the source of nourishment and comfort, a sign of impending puberty and perhaps the most unambiguous symbols of femininity and sexuality.

Whether you have breasts, or you know women who do, I'm sure you'll agree that breasts, with all their various sizes and shapes, are endlessly fascinating. Sadly, for some women, they are instead an endless source of self-consciousness, discomfort or loss. For these women, breast surgery can make an incalculable difference.

If they are your breasts and you want to change them for your own good reasons, then you should know that you have options. You should learn all you can about the procedure you want, the contra-indications and risks, and you should work with a top-notch surgical team. It's important to have realistic expectations and to realize that while computer-simulated results are helpful, they aren't a promise of those exact results.

Until I began to research cosmetic surgery for breasts, I was kind of snotty about it. I figured that most of the women who wanted breast implants were seeking double Ds to please a husband or attract a boyfriend. Although breast enlargement is the most common procedure, in truth it is more often women who want a more natural looking change, from an A-cup to a C for example. Breast enlargement is considered safe and so common it is a routine surgery these days and implants are safer than ever.

Breast enlargement is only part of the story. Breast reduction can help women with chronic back pain and sore shoulders as overly heavy breasts can cause bra straps to cut into tender flesh. Imagine carrying a five- or ten-pound bag of potatoes hanging from your neck all day, every day and you'll understand.

For some women, a breast lift, with or without implants, can restore the shape of the breasts after the effects of pregnancy, nursing, age and gravity. Why shouldn't we want to look and feel our best? After all, most women live into their 70s or 80s, and studies show that we are sexual beings our whole lives. For some women, a breast lift can improve her self-confidence and feelings of desirability.

Not all breast surgery is to enlarge, reduce or lift breasts. Some women want surgery to restore a breast after a mastectomy or other cancer treatment. Others want to correct a noticeable asymmetry. And breast surgery isn't limited to women. Men sometimes seek breast reduction, too.

Research convinced me that my early attitude against breast surgery was narrow-minded. After looking at hundreds of before and after photos, I saw many amazing transformations. I began to understand why cosmetic surgery was important for the women involved and realized that if they could afford the surgery, why shouldn't they have it? It's their life, their body.

Of course, just as an experienced surgeon and a top-notch facility are important for a good outcome, affordability is a factor. Typically, cosmetic surgery is not covered by insurance in the US unless it is for post-mastectomy reconstruction and the out-of-pocket expense is prohibitive for many women who might otherwise opt to have surgery. However, the cost of breast procedures vary from country to country, and Mexico offers some of the best options available today.

Cosmetic Surgery: Evaluating the Risks

Cosmetic surgery, like most surgeries, is relatively safe. However, like all surgeries, there is some risk of complications, even a slight risk of death. For example, according to the American Society of Anesthesiologist, anesthesia-related deaths occur 1 in 250,000 procedures in the US. However, doctors feel that even if the risk is slight, surgery should be considered carefully.

Many people are attracted to having cosmetic surgery in Mexico primarily because of the lower costs. The more popular of these are nose surgery, liposuction, breast enlargement/reduction, eyelid surgery, and facelifts. Each procedure poses some level of risk for a wide variety of complications in addition to the risk of death. This would be true wherever the surgery was performed.

Cosmetic surgery is a viable option for many people, particularly when someone has a facial malformation (for example, a clef palette) or need for reconstructive surgery such as breast reconstruction following a mastectomy as a treatment for breast cancer. However, for every patient seeking this kind of life-altering surgery, there is someone who wants a nose like Jennifer Lawrence's or bigger breasts. Is it worth taking a risk, however small, for improvements like these?

I am reminded of the risks involved because of a news story involving a beautiful, young (age 29) woman from Australia who died during cosmetic surgery in Mexico. She'd undertaken research on the doctor's website, had seen his professional memberships and read the recommendations and watched the videos. She felt confident there would be no problems. Sadly, she died on the operating table of a pulmonary embolism and acute pulmonary edema.

I don't know if this woman's death was related to malpractice or just bad luck, but there were some irregularities in her case and authorities are investigating a previous post-surgery death at the same practice the year before. But whatever the outcome of this investigation, it prompts me to remind readers of the following:

1. Are you in good general health? Elective surgery should almost always be avoided if you have a medical condition: diabetes, high blood pressure, blood clotting issues, heart problems, etc. Even if you are overweight and are seeking liposuction or bariatric surgery, you should be healthy before you consider surgery.

2. Cosmetic surgery can't make you young again. Yes, it may temporarily improve your looks, but we are all destined to age, if we are fortunate. Like a Hollywood actress with a face frozen by Botox injections, at a certain point, even with cosmetic surgery, people won't notice your attractiveness, but rather will notice how good you look for your age. You cannot escape aging.

3. Don't believe everything you read and see on a doctor or clinic's website. That content is not objective. It is carefully crafted to attract new patients. I am not saying that it is inaccurate. However, it may not tell the whole story.

4. Dig deeper. Investigate more than just the doctor's website. Are there complaints? Bad reviews? News stories? Search for these! Look at page 5 or 10 on Google, not just the first page.

5. Make sure that all of your questions are answered, and all your concerns are addressed when speaking to a doctor and his or her staff. Are you being rushed? Are they more focused on your payment than your well-being? If you are considering a particular doctor or clinic, ask for referrals that you can speak to and actually contact them.

6. Get a referral for a board certified surgeon in good standing from the actual medical board. In fact, it would be better to get three referrals, to review their credentials and experience and to speak to all three of them before deciding which one is best for you. [*See Medical Board Certification & Medical Specialties*]

These suggestions don't apply just to Mexico, but anywhere in the world where you might consider travel for surgery. To a remarkable degree, the medical care you will find in Mexico is good to superior, but even working with the world's best surgeon does not eliminate all risk. So, do what you can to reduce the risks and make sure the upside benefits are worth taking any risk.

Experimental & Non-Approved Treatments

Many healing techniques, modalities and medicines, now common in the rest of the world, were adopted long ago in Mexico and have been benefiting patients for years. This is just as true today and one of the gifts of the medical system of Mexico is that it is less restrictive about experimental medicine, giving hope and new possibilities to heal for those with serious illnesses, especially cancer.

Of course, as with any form of experimentation, not everything works as expected, and perhaps more than in the USA, Canada or the United Kingdom, the patient him or herself shoulders the responsibility for making life and death decisions regarding their own care. Malpractice insurance is uncommon in Mexico and neither you, nor your survivors, will have someone with deep pockets to sue.

The idea that a patient would sue a doctor for a bad outcome is ludicrous to Mexicans who are in general disbelief about the large awards given in the US. So, you need to do your own research, understand the treatment and calculate the risks carefully. Ask all the questions you need to ask to assure yourself that the treatment you are seeking is likely to be beneficial and make sure you discover what the downside is as well in case things don't go as planned.

Some of the therapies being used in Mexico were originally developed in the US, but the physicians involved were subsequently pressured to leave by repeated harassment, legal action or investigatory actions by medical authorities. Many found a new home in Mexico.

A number of the alternative cures for cancer used in Mexico have proven to be effective and even life-saving for individuals who have run out of approved options—the traditional surgery/radiation/chemotherapy routinely practiced in the US and Canada. This is all the more remarkable given that the typical cancer patient visiting Mexico for treatment is stage 4 and has already had all the chemo and radiation possible. Despite the lives being saved, the American Cancer Society questions many of the practices and therapies being offered in Mexico.

While we can give you information about treatments, and in some cases contact information, we cannot verify the validity of the claims made for these treatments, nor can we vouch for the qualifications of the practitioners. Although we strive to give you the best of the best, you will need to do your own research. [*See Appendix N: Alternative Medical Clinics in Mexico*]

Second opinions are always valuable too. For example, before you decide to seek alternative treatment for cancer, you may also want to consult with Ralph W. Moss PhD, a respected specialist who has many years of experience researching and writing about both standard mainstream and alternative treatments for cancer and who has visited many of the treatment clinics in Mexico.[39] Here is a free in-depth research paper by Dr. Moss entitled Tijuana Cancer Clinics in the Post-NAFTA Era. You'll need to register to download.[40]

Alternative Therapies in Mexico

Mexico, has become an international center for alternative therapies that are not available, at least affordably, in other parts of the world. Here is a list of some of the therapies currently practiced in Mexico. Some of the hospitals and clinics offering these treatments are in an appendix at the back of this book. [*See Appendix N: Alternative Medical Clinics in Mexico*] Listing these treatments does not guarantee their efficacy. Please review the disclaimer at the beginning of this book. [*See Disclaimer*]

Biomagnetic Cancer Therapy

Biomagnetic cancer therapy uses magnets on the body to promote self-healing. It repolarizes cancer cells and has anti-inflammatory effects, to reduce pain and discomfort. Biomagnetic therapy may also be used to treat chronic degenerative diseases.

Chelation Therapy

This is a treatment for acute mercury, iron (including in cases of thalassemia), arsenic, lead, uranium, plutonium and other forms of toxic metal poisoning. Depending on the agent and the type of poisoning, the chelating agent may be administered intravenously, intramuscularly, or orally. Chelation therapy is also used for treatment of coronary artery disease with recent study that shocked the traditional medical community by reducing the risk of cardiovascular events by 18%.[41]

Heberprot-P

This medicine, developed in Cuba, provides much needed help for diabetics facing the possible amputation of a foot. Currently there are 70,000 to 80,000 diabetics who become amputees every year in the US due to diabetic foot ulcers. Heberprot-P can reduce the relative risk by 75% and is therefore highly effective. There are clinics in Mexico devoted to this treatment (Mexico has an unusually high instance of diabetes), although with warming relations between the US and Cuba, it may soon not be necessary to seek treatment in Mexico.[42]

High Intensity Focused Ultrasound (HIFU)

High Intensity Focused Ultrasound (HIFU) is an experimental non-invasive, non-surgical ultrasound treatment that is intended to help patients with prostrate conditions retain sexual function and avoid other negative side effects of standard surgical procedures.[43]

Hyperthermia

This is an approach to treating tumors that induces a fever (or uses some other method) in order to raise the body temperature internally. It assumes that the tumor cells are less heat resilient than normal body cells are and that exposure to heat will kill cells and shrink tumors.

Ibogaine

Drug addiction, especially opiate addiction, has become an epidemic in the USA. According to the Centers for Disease Control there are over 2 million people in the USA addicted to opiates. There were over 16,000 deaths from overdosing on prescription opioids and over 8,000 deaths from heroin in 2013.[44] Opiate addiction is notoriously difficult to treat. Iboaine, a psychedelic substance from a West African plant, has shown promise as an experimental treatment for opiate withdrawl and along with conventional treatment such as a 2-step program, can help with kicking an opiate addiction. Illegal in the US, ibogaine treatment is available in Mexico.[45]

Immune Therapy

Active immunotherapies stimulate the body's own immune system to fight the disease. Passive immunotherapies do not rely on the body to attack the disease; but rather use immune system components (such as antibodies) made in the lab. This approach is sometimes referred to as a type of non-toxic cancer vaccine.

Insulin Potentiation Therapy

Insulin Potentiation Therapy, or IPT, can reduce the side effects of chemotherapy by lowering the dose of chemotherapy drugs needed. In IPT, a small amount of insulin is applied to open the glucose receptors in cancer cells. Chemotherapy drugs are then mixed with the glucose solution and applied directly to the cancer cells.

Integrative Medicine

Using a variety of techniques to deal with the physical, nutritional, psychotherapeutic and spiritual dimensions of an illness. Some of these practices do extensive testing and design protocols based on the unique needs of individual patients.

Medical Marijuana

Mexico has very strict drugs laws and an ongoing "War on Drugs." However, recent changes in the law allow very limited use of marijuana for medicinal use when prescribed by a physician for serious illnesses such as epilepsy. Do not assume that self-prescribed treatment will be tolerated, nor that local law-enforcement officials will be up-to-date on these changes in the law. At this time, if you go to a traditional medical doctor requesting medical marijuana or any narcotic medicine, it will be assumed that you are seeking the drug for recreational use and not medical treatment. Medical marijuana has only been approved for four individuals at this time.

Micronutrient Therapy

This is an approach to treating cancer and other chronic or degenerative diseases with vitamins and other nutrients. It is often part of an integrated approach to cancer treatment.

Oxygen, Ozone and Bio Oxidative Therapy

This therapy saturates the body or blood with oxygen in order to produce a hostile environment for viruses. Some use intravenous drips of medical grade hydrogen peroxide. Others use hyperbaric chambers to surround the patient with an oxygen-rich environment under pressure for a specified amount of time. Hyperbaric chambers are also used to treat deep-sea divers who are suffering from the "bends" and are commonly found in popular resort and diving areas on the coasts of Mexico.

Peptide and Protein Therapy

Different from traditional drugs, peptides occur naturally in the body. They are now being used in a therapeutic approach to treating a wide range of diseases from neurological diseases like Alzheimer's, brain injury, and dementia, to rheumatic conditions like arthritis and lupus. Claims for this approach include significant increase in the cognitive function of advanced Alzheimer's patients.

Rife Therapy

Rife cancer therapy is a non-invasive treatment that uses bio-frequency to treat cancer and other diseases. In rife cancer therapy, the skin is not broken and healthy tissues and cells are not damaged.

Stem Cell Therapy

This technique is useful in the treatment of Parkinson's disease, Alzheimer's disease, multiple sclerosis (MS), spinal cord injuries, stroke, burns, heart disease, diabetes, osteoarthritis, rheumatoid arthritis, degeneration of the liver, and correction of genetic disorders is common in Mexico. Stem cells obtained from a patient's own blood may be used. Stem cells harvested using a fertile egg, a technique that is outlawed in the US, is also performed in Mexico.[46]

Ultraviolet Light Therapy

Often used in conjunction with other blood treatments, blood is passed through a chamber that exposes it to immune-response boosting ultraviolet light.

Vitamin B17 (Laetrile)

Vitamin B17 is derived from natural food sources, most abundantly from seeds of plants from the *prunasin* family such as apricots and apples. It is sometimes used therapeutically as a cancer treatment and preventative, although it was banned by the FDA in the 1980s. It is that is controversial due to its potential toxicity and questions about its efficacy.[47]

Women's Health

In Mexico you will find all of the health services you would expect to find in the US and Canada including gynecologists, obstetricians, endocrinologists, and specialists in breast cancer and breast reconstruction. Birth control, in many forms, including birth control pills and condoms are widely available. While your specific brand may or may not be found in Mexico [*See Finding Your Medicine in Mexico*], you will undoubtedly find something chemically the same or similar and a doctor who specializes in women's health to help you.

Pregnancy & Childbirth

Pregnancy and childbirth in Mexico are honored events and you will find plenty of support and approval for pregnancy and childbirth in this highly family-oriented culture. In some parts of the country homebirth and midwifery are still practiced, although most children are born in hospitals these days. Some cities have hospitals or maternity centers that are devoted to delivering babies and maternal and infant care. In rural Mexico it is common for teens to marry and bear children. In fact, this is the norm. What is new in Mexican culture is single motherhood.

The most serious health problem for infants currently is the threat of the Zika virus to unborn babies. [*See Zika Virus*] It is vitally important that women of childbearing age learn to protect themselves from infection and if possible, to avoid the regions where mosquitoes and the diseases they may carry are the biggest problems.

For mothers-to-be, the rising rates of pregnancies that are delivered by C-section is a health concern. There will always be some instances where C-section is absolutely required, but sometimes it is planned for the doctor's or mother's convenience, and sometimes it is the result of impatience on the part of obstetricians.

Increased Rates of C-sections

Increasing rates of C-sections is part of a worldwide trend in developed countries and seems to be a particularly popular in Mexico. C-sections are unusually high in physician assisted hospital births. While reliable statistics are difficult to find, the numbers sometimes cited of C-sections as a percentage of overall births are shockingly high—up to 80 percent for example.

Birth is frequently a slow and painful process. C-sections are a high-billing "solution" that frees a doctor's time for other pursuits and foreshortens what some patients perceive to be unnecessary suffering. Many mothers are not aware of the increased maternal mortality associated with C-sections.

While these attitudes are not exclusively those of obstetricians and pregnant women in Mexico (for example, scheduled C-sections are becoming increasingly popular in the USA), slow vaginal deliveries are the way nature intended babies to be born and many studies show that natural vaginal births are much safer for both the mother and child. Recovery for the mother is longer and more painful post C- section and reduces the chances of subsequent vaginal birth.

Of course, after the fact there is often a "reason" given for the more invasive medical intervention, even when labor is progressing normally, the baby is in good position, the mother coping well, the birth weight of the baby in the normal range and no other high-risk factors are present.

The best way to avoid unnecessary C-section is to ask potential obstetricians what percentage of their deliveries result in C-section. If the percentage is higher than 20% it falls outside of the rate the World Health Organization feels is appropriate. Keep looking.

A good source of information and referrals to obstetricians who can help you achieve a safe and natural birth is the La Leche League where mothers who have a commitment to respecting the natural processes of birth and breastfeeding will tend to gather. [*See La Leche League*]

You may also want to investigate the use of a midwife since childbirth is not a disease and a well-trained and experienced midwife or nurse midwife will tend to be more patient with the natural process of birth. You will want to make certain any midwife you choose has an emergency back-up plan. But if you have no high-risk factors, this might be a reasonable alternative to a rushed and risky delivery by an allopathic physician.

The over-use of C-section deliveries is something that the medical community in Mexico needs to address. It profoundly affects the safety of childbirth for Mexicans and their children. It is also a major factor for young expat families who are deciding whether or not to have their children born in Mexico.

Breastfeeding

Breastfeeding is widely practiced in Mexico where it is considered a natural and normal maternal act. Unlike the US where women who feed their infants in public are often treated with scorn and where many breastfeeding women feel they must hide in a bathroom, it is not unusual to see women feeding infants quite openly in public places in Mexico: on the bus, in the park, in restaurants. An exposed breast generates no comments, no glares and women are not ashamed of feeding their children. Mexico sets a good example

Infants in Mexico tend to be held in arms or in a sling close to the body rather than pushed in a stroller. Strollers are nearly useless on cobble streets or where there are no sidewalks, although you do see them being used in large cities. The close physical bond of being held close and breastfed may be why babies and young children seem to be quieter and calm than their northern counterparts.

La Leche League

The La Leche League is an international organization that helps women get started with breastfeeding through local gatherings and coaches. In Mexico it is called *La Liga de La Leche* and you can find a local chapter on their website.[48] If you are pregnant or have a new baby, we recommend you attend even if your Spanish is poor. You can learn most of what you need by demonstration and being part of the community of new mothers will be helpful to you and your infant. You will find a list of the chapters in Mexico on *La Liga de La Leche's* website in the endnote above.

Contacting the La Leche League, attending gatherings and social networking can be a very good source of medical referrals, especially obstetricians and pediatricians.

Emergency Contraception

"Morning after" pills, sold under the name "Plan B" in the US, are available at *farmacias* in Mexico under the name *Cerciora-t (Levonorgestrel)*. Two pills, (0.75mg ea.) are sold at a cost of about 100 pesos. Planned Parenthood offers advice about using emergency contraception.[49]

Abortion Medicines

Mexican pharmacies on the border have become popular destinations for those from the USA seeking abortion medicines. One of the two medications used in a medically induced abortion— misoprostol— is available as an ulcer medication in some parts of Mexico without a prescription under the name Cytotec.[50] Use of this medicine alone (it is typically used in the USA in combination with another medication) is not considered a safe, nor effective way to induce abortion.

Just because you can buy these pills in Mexico does not mean it will be safe for you to talk about using them, to use them without medical supervision or use them outside of Mexico City. To do so could result in serious medical and/or legal consequences.[51] Women have been prosecuted in Mexico for going to a hospital showing the symptoms of attempted abortion. This includes hemorrhage from a medically induced abortion. You do not want to have to make a choice between bleeding to death and going to jail.

Abortion Rights

As in many predominantly Catholic countries, abortion is widely frowned upon, and in fact illegal in most of Mexico. Despite the prohibition, an estimated 4.2 million women throughout Latin America and the Caribbean risk death each year as a result of illegal abortions. Mexico has sought a humane solution by making Mexico City a place where women can obtain safe, legal and free or low-cost abortions in public health facilities. But ONLY in Mexico City.

Legal abortions are not only humane; they are cost effective. The average cost of a legal abortion in Mexico City is between $79 and $143 USD (and often free for indigent women), whereas the cost to treat the complications of an illegal abortion range from $600 to over $2000 USD per patient.

Outside of Mexico City, abortion is only permitted in cases of rape, but according to Human Rights Watch, at least 130 women have been sentenced in Mexico for seeking or providing legal abortions. Therefore, it is recommended that you not even discuss abortion with a doctor outside of Mexico City.

Fertility Treatments

In Vitro Fertilization (IVF)

Approximately ten percent of couples have difficulty conceiving or bringing a fetus to full-term. So while the condition of infertility is hardly rare, for the couples involved it can be a devastating and highly personal plight. Fortunately, we live in a day and age when a wide range of treatment options are available, although frequently not affordable to those who need it most.

Mexico, perhaps uniquely, extends heartfelt compassion to an infertile couple or individuals who are seeking to become pregnant. Because family life is so important in Mexico, there is good treatment and care for both Mexican citizens and foreigners who need medical support. This is a blessing because many necessary and costly treatments are not covered by insurance in the United States. (Nor are they covered by IMSS, the largest insurer in Mexico.)

While there are no guarantees in life, there are many babies that have been conceived in Mexico and brought successfully to term. The fertility support websites in the US and Canada are full of stories about people visiting Mexico for care and you may want to connect with others who can share their experiences with you. One of the largest and most respected organizations for people coping with infertility is Resolve, the National Infertility Association. There are also many websites offering helpful community forums such as Fertile Thoughts.

In an appendix at the end of this book you will find a list of hospitals that are permitted by health authorities in Mexico to perform those procedures that involve the harvesting of eggs or sperm and the implanting of embryos—the most invasive of fertility procedures. [*See Appendix O: Fertility Treatment Centers*] Therefore, these facilities are also the most likely to offer a full range of fertility treatments. Many of them have websites in English for the benefit of those who are considering the option of traveling to Mexico in order to fulfill their dream of having a child.

Surrogacy

Until fairly recently, India was the only option for those seeking to create a family through surrogacy. However, the gulf state of Tabasco in Mexico is the only state currently that allows surrogacy, theoretically on a non-commercial basis. Regretfully, the state legislature also voted to ban this option for both gay men and foreigners. However, for Mexican women ages 35 to 40 who can prove they are medically unable to bear a child, surrogacy is a possibility in Tabasco.

Surrogacy for foreigners has not work out in most of the world where it has been practiced in the past. Places where it was once legal, but now not, include India, Thailand and now Mexico.

Problems with Altitude

Altitude illness is not something people typically think of when visiting or living in Mexico. While altitude can become a significant issue for a small few people, for most of us it's a matter of taking time to acclimatize.

If you're planning to visit or live in one of the popular destinations in the central highlands of Mexico, you'll be going to a high-altitude zone. The more popular destinations at altitude include:

- Mexico City: 2,250 meters (7,350 feet)
- Guadalajara: 1,560 meters (5,108 feet)
- Querétaro: 1,860 meters (6,100 feet)
- San Miguel de Allende: 1,900 meters (6,233 feet)
- Cuernavaca: 1,510 meters (5,000 feet)
- Tepoztlán: 1,710 meters (5,600 feet)
- Puebla: 2,135 meters (7,005 feet)
- Guanajuato: 2,012 meters (6,600 feet)
- Oaxaca: 1,585 meters (5,200 feet)
- San Cristóbal de las Casas: 2,200 meters (7,200 feet)

While these cities are known for their idyllic climate (typically characterized by warm sunny days, and cool nights), they are also situated at altitudes that might prove challenging for a short while after you arrive. Considering the elevation of a place is especially important for travelers with asthma or other breathing problems, and Mexico City is particularly challenging for those with breathing difficulties between December and April, when the combination of the altitude and trapped air pollution can make the capital's air quite uncomfortable.

The symptoms of altitude sickness can take two or three days to make themselves apparent and may include:

- Headaches
- Loss of appetite
- Dizziness or nausea
- Fatigue
- Sleeplessness
- Shortness of breath

Related information about altitude illness later in this book, offers more technical information for climbers with tips and advice to help you acclimatize to higher altitudes. [*See Altitude Illness*] It can take up to a week for your body to fully adjust.

Altitude sickness is rarely fatal at altitudes below 11,000 feet (3,500 meters), and on average Mexico's colonial cities are situated at an elevation of some 6,000 feet above sea level. The summit of Mexico's highest mountain, Pico de Orizaba, peaks at 5,636 m (18,500 feet)—and even that is well below the so-called 'death zone' of 8,000 meters: the height at which oxygen levels are too low to sustain human life. Nonetheless, anyone planning to undertake mountaineering expeditions in Mexico should come well prepared.

For a small few people, even altitudes over a couple of thousand feet may cause health problems. If your symptoms are more serious, seek lower elevation (head to the coast) and seek immediate medical attention. Medical professionals may administer oxygen or Acetazolamide (Diamox) to stimulate breathing. If you have had altitude sickness before, consider asking your doctor for this medication as a preventative measure.

For some people, especially runners and other endurance athletes, Mexico's high elevation areas are exactly what they are looking for, and many runners preparing for international competition train in the mountains around Mexico City.

If you are looking for a "kick your butt" training challenge, try the 1,200 foot run-climb to the mountain pyramid "El Tepozteco," in Tepoztlán, Morelos. As *Modern Hiker's* website puts it, "There aren't too many places where you can find a trail that will kick your butt with elevation gain, bring you to the ruins of a 500-year-old religious complex, and drop you off right next to a market filled with unbelievably delicious hand-made food…"

Volcanoes & Earthquakes

You will see them all over Mexico City: painted green squares or circles, usually with arrows pointing inward. Usually they are on the sidewalk or perhaps in the middle or a parking lot. Sometimes they are in the middle of the street. These are called "puntos de reunion" (meeting points). They are the place where people can gather during an earthquake, a safe spot in an open place unlikely to be hit with falling debris.

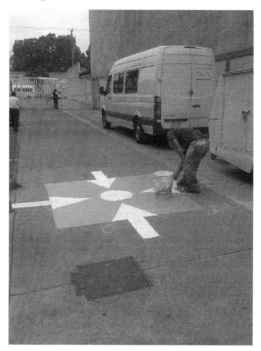

Punto de reunion

In 1985 a major earthquake hit Mexico City and as many as 10,000 people were killed, primarily due to inadequate construction that flattened during the quake Since then, considerable effort and investment has been made in construction improvements and safety regulations including the puntos.

Mexico is a volcanically active area. Both Colima in Jaliso and Popocatepetl in the states of Puebla and Morelos are considered active and occasionally disrupt air traffic with outpourings of volcanic ash. However, major eruptions are nearly impossible to predict. If and when a volcano erupts (and there are dozens of them in Mexico), the damage and disruption can be widespread and there are evacuations. However, the likelihood of an earthquake is greater than an eruption and if you are not from a seismically active area, you may not know what to do if the ground starts to move beneath your feet.

If you experience an earthquake—

- If you are indoors, it is better to stay there and get under a desk or table or stand next to an interior wall. Avoid exterior walls, heavy furniture, glass, fireplaces and appliances (kitchens are a bad place to be).
- If you are in an office building, do not use the elevator and stay away from exterior walls and windows.
- If you are driving, move carefully out of traffic and stop. Avoid parking under or on bridges or overpasses. If possible, stay clear of traffic lights, trees, light poles, signs and power lines. When driving, watch for road hazards.
- If you are in a mountain region, there is a potential for landslides. If you are near the ocean, get to high ground since tsunamis are possible with large earthquakes.
- If you are in a crowded public place, do not rush for the exit. You are more likely to be hurt by panic, so just stay low and cover your head and neck with your arms and hands.

Hurricanes

Seasonal storms are not infrequent in Mexico. The season for tropical storms typically starts mid May and continues to the end of October (although the few tropical storms that actually become hurricanes happen in July, August or September). In general, the Atlantic seaboard of Mexico is more likely to experience hurricanes than the Pacific.

If you are planning a beach vacation during the July-September timeframe, it is a good idea to purchase travel insurance and keep an eye on the weather. Many coastal hotels have been built specially to withstand topical storms or even full-force hurricanes. However, in the most serious instances you may need to be evacuated. This happens rarely, but evacuating early and moving inland is a much better option than risking life and limb and experiencing the terror those who choose to hunker down in a hotel room during a hurricane often experience.

If you live in a coastal area of Mexico, you need to have a preparedness plan including safety equipment (flash lights, radio, generator, etc.) and the supplies needed for several days without electricity including food and water. You too should be prepared to evacuate if a serious hurricane is expected to make landfall near you.

It is customary for everyone in Mexico to pitch in with needed food and supplies during a disaster. Staple foods like rice, beans and canned goods and personal care products such as toilet paper, soap, toothbrushes and toothpaste, combs and brushes, and blankets and towels are usually accepted. There is often a list of needed items broadcast on radio and television or handed out at the local Red Cross.

Goods are typically collected at a local Red Cross facility and trucked to the disasters. Volunteers will receive your donations, sort everything and prepare the goods for shipment. Mexico may have many poor citizens, but when it comes to helping in a disaster, everyone gets involved and generously donates resources and time. If you reside in Mexico, you should too.

Medical Emergencies

As of Jan. 2017, the universal emergency number in Mexico is 911. Please be aware that even though this number should work on cell phones, cell phone service is unreliable in places. If you are using a cell phone from outside of Mexico, make certain it works in Mexico by testing. (Do not test by calling 911.)

If you are on a toll road, there is typically an emergency number printed on your receipt for emergency help (typically for CAPUFE). This is the number to call for car accidents, but they may be able to call for medical help in an emergency.

Almost by definition, no one expects an emergency. And because we don't expect them, we are often ill prepared. Even in our home countries we seldom think about what we'd do beyond picking up the phone and dialing 911. Ambulances are available in nearly every population center in the USA and Canada and most communities have paramedics and hospital emergency rooms available 24/7 every day of the year. Yes, it may be expensive — maybe even prohibitively expensive. Yes, you may have to wait for treatment, perhaps for hours, but emergency treatment is widely available.

In Mexico things are different, often very different than they are back where we expats came from. Not necessarily worse or better, but it is easy to be taken by surprise because we tend to make assumptions based on our life experiences. I know because this is what happened to me. I had a medical emergency and despite having a lot more knowledge than the average foreigner about medical care in Mexico (after all, I've researched extensively and have written a book on the subject) I made some basic assumptions that just didn't pan out. Here's what happened.

It was Christmas Day and during the night I became ill. By 4:00 am it was clear that I needed to see a doctor as soon as possible. I was able to walk so I didn't require an ambulance, and there wasn't an ambulance service nearby in any case. My partner was able to drive me from the rural area where I lived to the nearest city, about 45 minutes away.

We headed to the small private hospital that was owned and run by my personal physician, someone I trusted. Although the hospital has only 13 beds (common for private hospitals in Mexico), it does have a small emergency room and we expected to be received there by the physician on duty. I'd been treated there uneventfully before and so had my partner.

Navidad, (Christmas) is one of the most important holidays in Mexico. It is a time when families frequently go on vacation and nearly all businesses close. Even Mexico City, typically teeming with people on streets lined with bustling shops and filled with traffic, will be shuttered and vacant — a virtual ghost town.

So, the much-smaller city we'd driven to was desolate and we were able to get to the hospital in record time. What we hadn't anticipated was that when we got there, the hospital would be closed. Completely. Metal shutters covered the entrance. Evidently there had been no in-patients, so they simply closed the doors and all the staff was able to take time off for the holiday. Who would have thought?

Fortunately, I wasn't dealing with a life-or-death crisis. If I had been, I might not be writing this story. However, it was scary to find ourselves alone on the street, at night, in a city that was deserted without an immediate plan for what to do next.

My husband was familiar with the city and after several tense minutes of wandering aimlessly, he had a notion about where to go. Before too long we were at the gates of a larger private hospital where a large, brightly lit sign suggested it might be open. It was a relief when the electronic gate opened and an attendant waved us into the nearly empty parking lot. (Evidently, everyone in Mexico stays healthy for Christmas.)

Within a few moments we walked into a spotless, bright, ultra-modern and well-equipped emergency room and saw a doctor immediately. After all of my vitals were taken, the doctor made a diagnosis and prescribed a medication, all handled with an admirable level of compassion, efficiency and professionalism, we were given the bill: 300 pesos, or roughly $22.50 USD. We were directed to a nearby 24-hour pharmacy where the medicine was obtained for 50 pesos ($3.70 USD) and soon we were heading home.

The problems we encountered that night were not Mexico's issues. They were mine. I simply wasn't prepared with the knowledge of the culture and the local services I needed to have. For example, I now know that public hospitals tend to be open on holidays, whereas private hospitals, as you can see, may or may not be.

But there's a lot more to know in order to get the best possible care in Mexico. As of the beginning of 2017, the national number for emergencies everywhere is 911. However, you need to also have local emergency numbers: the numbers of both public and private ambulance services, where the nearest public and private hospitals are and the best routes to get there, the phone numbers of the hospitals so you can call from a cell phone en route and, as I discovered, information about whether they are open for important holidays or not. [*See Uncertain Emergency Response*]

Insects Can Be Serious Health Hazards

Mosquitoes

Where I live, at high altitude, mosquitoes can usually be avoided by closing unscreened doors and windows in the evening and early morning hours when these flying insects typically feed. For houses without screens, a bed net is highly suggested, not only for comfort, but to avoid the transmission of insect-borne illnesses. Unless you are roughing it in rural or coastal areas, that should be enough. Or so I thought.

Then there was that sunny afternoon I spent celebrating *Navidad* (Christmas) at a fiesta in our *jardin* (garden or yard), breaking a piñata and lighting sparklers with the kids. Later that night it was clear that I'd been badly bitten, all below the knees, yet I had not seen, nor heard, nor felt a single mosquito. After a night of tortured itching (and scratching) I made a visit to a doctor both for treatment and to discover what sort of insect had assaulted me.

The doctor explained that the culprits were a variety of mosquito that hid in the grass and fed during the day. She told me that she uses insect repellant containing DEET every day and so should I, and that I should also wear clothing that covered my skin.

While to many travelers and expats this may seem excessive, I suggest that you read the IAMAT section in this book and make note of the sheer number of serious diseases that are conveyed by mosquito. [*See IAMAT Travel Advice for Mexico*] Fortunately this section also offers a good deal of advice for how to avoid being bitten by mosquitoes. [*See Preventing insect bites*]

One of the most serious of the mosquito-borne diseases is the Zika virus. As of January 2017, over 7,000 people in Mexico have been infected with this virus. This is part of a worldwide epidemic. Even the USA has had over 5,000 cases in the same timeframe. Zika is considered dangerous for both men and women, and that goes double for pregnant women and their unborn children and women of child-bearing age. Avoiding exposure to mosquitoes (and having sex with someone who has been infected) are the key to prevention until a vaccine is widely available. [*See Zika Virus*]

Scorpions

Regretfully, I also have firsthand experience with scorpions as well as mosquitoes. I just looked at a map that shows the range of scorpions and it looks like they are all over the USA, Mexico, Central and South America. There are even some in Canada. Like the Southwestern US, there are plenty of them where I live in the mountains of central Mexico.

The scorpions where I live tend to be small and reddish, maybe 3 to 6 centimeters (about an inch or an inch and a half) typically, and our local variety isn't considered life threatening. But they do end up in the house, and it is recommended that you shake out towels and clothing before using them and shake out your shoes.

In my house they seem to like the kitchen best, and sometimes there will be one in the sink when I wake up. So, I should have known better than to reach into the sink to remove a couple of plates I'd left there overnight. Ouch! There was a sharp burning pain on my first knuckle. I shook my hand and looked, but there wasn't much to see. It just hurt like hell. I didn't even have to lift the plates to know what had happened. In a moment of carelessness, I'd been stung by a scorpion. Now I'd have to take quick action.

While there are almost 2,000 species of scorpions, only 30 or 40 have venom strong enough to kill a person. However, the greater threat is having an allergic reaction and ensuing anaphylactic shock. So it is best to act conservatively and get immediate medical attention. And because scorpion stings are fairly common where I lived, I was prepared with an antihistamine that I took immediately. (The doctors who treated me pointed out, the antihistamine won't really solve the potential problem, but it can delay the effects of an allergic reaction long enough to get you to more serious treatment, so I always keep them on hand.)

The town I lived in was so small that it didn't have a hospital. We could have made the trip to the city that's about 30 or 40 minutes away, but we decided against that in favor of a small public clinic that we'd seen many times before but never been inside. Our reasoning was that they probably get a lot of scorpion stings there, and we were right.

We knew that the clinic probably had some government affiliation, but it was only later that we learned it was run by the federal government as part of the "Seguro Popular" system that offers a range of medical care for those who aren't covered under the IMSS, ISSSTE or other medical care system in Mexico.

One of the complaints you sometimes hear about the public system is that it is crowded, that there are long waits. But when my husband and I entered the modern building in mid-afternoon, it was basically empty. Within minutes I was under observation and warned that I might be for an hour or more until it was clear I wasn't reacting to the venom. Every ten or fifteen minutes a staff member checked on me, asking me to report even the slightest changes in my nose, throat or breathing.

Mostly, I had nothing to report. But then, after about an hour I felt a very strong sensation in my nasal passages. It was like that intense feeling you get just before a sneeze, only this wasn't followed by sneezing. I told the doc and I was immediately taken to a bright, clean ward and told to lie on the bed. In less than a minute I was given a vial of anti-venom through a vein in my hand. Other than the small prick of the needle, I felt no pain, no sensation at all. The nose tickles stopped and I was soon on my way.

Because of the research I've done on the cost of medical care, I was aware that that little vial of potentially lifesaving anti-venom I'd received would typically cost about $100 USD at any private hospital in Mexico. People sometimes need more that one vial. The doctors that treated me told me about a baby they treated who required 11 vials.

The anti-venom I received was developed in Mexico. It has been used worldwide to save the lives of scorpion sting victims. Remarkably, that same vial of anti-venom would cost between $7,900 and $12,467 USD in the USA.

It sounds like I'm making that up doesn't it? I'm not. Here's a story about a woman who was treated for a scorpion sting in Phoenix. It took 2 vials and she was billed a whopping $83,046 USD. Her insurance company only picked up $57,509.[52]

Ironic isn't it? The US medical system is so broken that even someone with insurance is left to pay $25,000 USD out of pocket for a treatment that costs $100 USD in Mexico. Because it was considered emergency care, my treatment at *Seguro Popular* was free. I was not only grateful to be alive, but unburdened by backbreaking debt. Perhaps you understand now why I often feel such abundant gratitude for the medical care I receive in Mexico.

Brown Recluse Spiders

I am happy to report that I have not, to my knowledge, encountered a brown recluse spider. Normally found in the central and southern USA, these arachnoids arrived in Mexico in 2015 and a number of bites have been reported.

The tiny brown recluse spiders (only about 1 x 1.5 cms) are sometimes called the violin spider because they have markings on their back that resemble a violin. They are brown in color, but the shade may vary, and the fine hair that covers their abdomen gives it a velvety appearance. They have six eyes arranged in a semi-circle of three pairs.

Although they are so toxic that their bite kills over 200,000 people worldwide each year—and there is no antidote—90% of bites heal, often without medical attention. The symptoms include fever, nausea, sweating, itching, chills and a general feeling of discomfort or sickness.

Typically, the brown recluse spider only bites when disturbed and is found in dark, secluded places and at night (it is nocturnal). It is a good idea not to put your hands into places you cannot see. If you are bitten, apply ice and get immediate medical attention. Do not use your mouth to suck out the poison.

International Health Support

International Association for Medical Assistance to Travelers (IAMAT)

IAMAT is a non-profit organization whose mission for fifty years has been to provide impartial and accurate travel health advice. They coordinate an international network of qualified medical practitioners to assist travelers in need of emergency medical care during their trip.

Supported by donations, IAMAT provides its members referrals to local doctors and hospitals all over the world and a number of other benefits. Their popular lists of clinics and doctors around the world are revised annually and include a section for IAMAT-affiliated mental-health practitioners.

IAMAT, in the interest of providing support for our readers, has given us permission to reprint their travel information about Mexico. You can repay their kindness by joining IAMAT, making a donation and taking advantage of all the benefits of membership.[53]

International Society of Travel Medicine (ISTM) [54]

ISTM advances the specialty of travel medicine. The organization is comprised of 1,900 members in 53 countries who are committed to the promotion of healthy and safe travel. Members of ISTM include physicians, nurses and public health professionals from academia, government and the private sector.

ISTM maintains a directory of health-care professionals with expertise in travel medicine in almost 50 countries worldwide. They currently have only three member listings in Mexico: in Distrito Federal, Jalisco and Querétaro. You can visit here: International Society of Travel Medicine Clinic Directory.

International Medical Referrals

If you have a chronic illness you may find that there is a support organization that can put you in touch with specialists who treat patients with that particular disease all over the world. Although there are too many possibilities to list them here, you are probably already aware of the major organizations for your illness, if one exists. If not, an online search may provide this information.

Here is an example of the kind of support we are talking about. A person with Inflammatory Bowel Disease (IBD) might find a resource on About.com.[55] In turn, this page refers viewers to a number of organizations including the Society of Laparoendoscopic Surgeons, which has an international membership and lists two members in Mexico.[56] These physicians are highly likely to be able to offer either direct treatment of referrals to others who may be able to help.

IAMAT Travel Advice for Mexico

[Editor's Note: IAMAT uses British spellings in their publications and those have been retained in this following material.]

Preventing insect bites

During your travels you may encounter all types of insects, some of which are harmless while others can carry disease. Mosquitoes, ticks, bees, wasps, hornets, blackflies, spiders, and ants may be mild annoyances, but one small bite can have serious implications on your health.

Practicing meticulous and consistent insect bite avoidance is one of the most important things travellers can do to prevent illness and spreading infectious diseases. Of the common arthropod-borne diseases encountered by travellers, only Malaria and Japanese Encephalitis can be prevented by medication and a vaccine, respectively.

Here are 3 things to consider:

- You may not know that you have been bitten. Some insects like the Anopheles Malaria mosquito don't buzz and don't leave a welt after feeding.
- Depending on your body's tolerance, you may not develop hives, welts, itchy or burning skin – all signs indicating that you were bitten.
- If you were bitten by a disease-carrying insect, you may be asymptomatic, meaning you do not show any symptoms of the illness. Sometimes, you may even have a mild form of the illness and may think that you just have a flu or a cold, or even an unrelated skin rash.

Learn about insect behaviour

First, find out if, and exactly where, illnesses transmitted by insects are occurring at your destination. You may discover that there is no outbreak in the area where you're staying.

Second, learn about the insect's behaviour. This will help you better understand whether your travel, destination and activities have an element of risk or not.

- What is their habitat? Do they prefer the indoors, outdoors, or both?
- When are they most active, during the day or night? What are their peak biting times?
- Are they present year-round or do they have seasonal cycles?
- Do they live in urban, suburban, or rural areas?
- Are they capable of carrying illnesses transmitted to humans? If so, which ones?

Use complementary methods

For optimal protection, use multiple methods of insect-bite prevention – mainly through skin protection, clothing protection, and proper use of a bed net.

1. The following are physical barriers that you can use to prevent any insect from coming close to you in the first place.

- Wear light-coloured, loose-fitting, long clothing (cotton and linen) as much as possible.
- Don't use scented soaps, shampoos, deodorants, perfumes or after-shaves.
- Ensure that all door and window screens do not have tears or holes and that they are tightly fitted.
- Cover any food, drinks, compost and garbage.
- Always wear shoes, both indoors and outdoors.
- Sleep or rest under an insecticide-treated bed net.

2. Use chemical barriers like repellent and insecticide to prevent mosquito, tick, sandfly or blackfly bites.

- Use a spray, lotion, towelette, or liquid repellent containing 20-30% DEET or 20% Picaridin on exposed skin. Apply according to manufacturer's directions to ensure optimal protection. Re-apply on shorter times if you find that you are starting to get bitten. Note that repellents destroy items containing crystal or plastics so be careful if you wear jewellery or glasses.
- Treat clothing, shoes, boots, and gear with permethrin that kills insects on contact. Note that this product is not commercially available in Canada, but you can obtain it online through major US retailers. Do not use permethrin directly on your skin.
- Consider spraying your home or room with an insecticide. Note that some insects such as mosquitoes and bed bugs are becoming increasingly resistant to insecticides.
- When using repellents on children, check the manufacturer's directions. Talk to your doctor or travel health provider about using a repellent if you're travelling with an infant to an area with high risk of mosquito-transmitted illnesses. To further protect your child, ensure that they wear long light-coloured, loose-fitting clothing, cover their carrier with tight-fitting mosquito netting or place them under an insecticide-treated net when playing or resting.

A note on repellents and sunscreens

- Apply sunscreen first and repellent second. Allow the sunscreen to penetrate the skin for 20 minutes before using repellent. Note that this could reduce the efficacy of the sunscreen, so it's best to reapply often or wear long clothing.

Myth busting

It's important to use proven methods mentioned above, especially if you're travelling to areas with risk of illnesses transmitted by insects. There is no evidence that the following products protect you against insect-borne illnesses.

- Combined sunscreen and repellent lotions
- Citronella-based plants, coils, or candles
- Vitamin B1 or garlic
- Ultrasonic products, electrocuting devices, odour-infused traps
- Repellent-containing wristbands, ankle bands or neckbands

How to treat insect bites and stings

- If you have a skin reaction that includes hives, itching, red patches or a burning sensation, consider applying hydrocortisone cream 1% or a natural skin balm to relieve itching. To reduce hives, take a non-sedating antihistamine.
- If the site of the bite or sting swells, is very painful, and develops blisters, seek medical attention immediately.
- If you have a past history of life-threatening allergic reactions such as anaphylactic shock where you can't breathe or your throat swells, use an epinephrine auto-injector. Ensure that your travel companions know how to use one and seek medical care as soon as possible.

More about insect-avoidance tips

Mosquitoes

- Get rid of any containers or items holding water inside and outside a building.
- Sleep under an insecticide-treated bed net if you're going to an area with risk of Malaria or Japanese Encephalitis. For maximum protection, find out if you need anti-malarial medications or if the Japanese Encephalitis vaccine is recommended for your trip.

Ticks

- When hiking in wooded areas, tuck pants into socks, stay in the middle of the trail and avoid tall grasses and shrubs.
- Carefully examine your clothing, gear, and pets for ticks before entering a dwelling.
- Regularly check your body for ticks and promptly remove using tweezers by grasping the tick's head and mouth parts as much as possible and by pulling perpendicular from the skin.

- Thoroughly disinfect the bite site with soap and water or alcohol. If travelling in an endemic area, save the tick in a zip-lock bag or container to have it analyzed through your healthcare practitioner.

Sandflies

- This insect is active at night so it's best to avoid outdoor activities from dusk to dawn in risk areas.
- Sleep under an insecticide-treated bed net or air conditioned room.

Triatominae

- This nocturnal insect (also known as the kissing bug, 'vinchuca' in Spanish, or 'barbeiro' in Portuguese) is responsible for Chagas in the USA, Mexico, Central America and South America. Sleep under an insecticide-treated bed net.

Bed bugs

- This insect can be a traveller's worst nightmare and is becoming increasingly resistant to insecticides. If you get a bed bug infestation, it will cost you money, derail your travel plans, and may cause mental anguish. Bed bugs are known to carry pathogens that can cause human illnesses although whether they actively transmit them is still inconclusive. To prevent bed bug bites, see the Tip Sheet. [57]

Recommended Vaccinations:

Routine Immunizations

Your trip is a good occasion for a reminder to keep your routine immunizations updated. The following vaccinations are recommended for your protection and to prevent the spread of infectious diseases. World Immunization Chart [58]

Tetanus, Diphtheria, Pertussis, Measles, Mumps, Rubella, Polio should be reviewed and updated if necessary.

Note: Many of these vaccine preventable illnesses are making a resurgence due to non-vaccination, incomplete vaccination, and waning immunity. It is important to keep your routine immunization up-to-date.

Seasonal influenza vaccination is recommended for all travellers over 6 months of age, especially for children, pregnant women, persons over 65, and those with chronic health conditions such as asthma, diabetes, lung disease, heart disease, immune-suppressive disorders, and organ transplant recipients.

Note: In the northern hemisphere the flu season typically runs from November to April, from April to October in the southern hemisphere, and year-round in the tropics. If the flu vaccine is not available at the time of departure, contact your doctor or travel health clinic regarding influenza anti-viral protection.

Pneumococcal vaccine is recommended for persons over the age of 65 and persons of any age suffering from cardiovascular disease, diabetes, renal disorders, liver diseases, sickle cell disease, asplenia, or immuno-suppressive disorders.

Hepatitis A

Description

The Hepatitis A virus (HAV) is primarily transmitted from person to person via the fecal-oral route and through contaminated water and food - such as shellfish, and uncooked vegetables or fruit prepared by infected food handlers.

Risk

The virus is present worldwide, but the level of prevalence depends on local sanitary conditions. HAV circulates widely in populations living in areas with poor hygiene infrastructure. In these areas, persons usually acquire the virus during childhood when the illness is asymptomatic (but still infective to others) or mild, and end up developing full immunity. Large outbreaks in these countries are rare. In contrast, a large number of non-immune persons are found in highly industrialized countries where community wide outbreaks can occur when proper food handling or good sanitation practices are not maintained including in daycare centres, prisons, or mass gatherings.

Symptoms

In many cases, the infection is asymptomatic (persons do not exhibit symptoms). Those with symptoms will usually get ill between 15 to 50 days after becoming infected. Symptoms include malaise, sudden onset of fever, nausea, abdominal pain, and jaundice after a few days. The illness can range from mild to severe lasting from one to two weeks or for several months. Severe cases can be fatal especially in older persons. Most infections are asymptomatic in children under six years of age, but infants and children can continue to shed the virus for up to six months after being infected, spreading the infection to others. Many countries are now including vaccination against Hepatitis A in their childhood vaccination schedules.

Prevention

Practice good personal hygiene, including washing your hands frequently and thoroughly, drink boiled or bottled water, eat well cooked foods, and peel your own fruits.

Vaccination

Recommended for all travellers over 1 year of age.

There are two inactivated vaccines available in Canada and the USA, including a combined Hepatitis A and Hepatitis B vaccine. A combined Hepatitis A and Typhoid Fever vaccine is also available in Canada and Europe. Hepatitis A vaccines confer long term protection and can be given in accelerated schedules. Discuss your options with your healthcare provider if you cannot finish the series prior to your departure. Immune Globulin may be recommended for some last-minute travellers.

Typhoid Fever

Vaccination is recommended when going outside the areas usually visited by tourists such as travelling extensively in the interior of the country (e.g. trekkers, hikers), for persons on working assignments in remote areas, or travellers going to visit family and relatives for extended periods of time. It may also be recommended for travellers who use antacid therapy.

Description

Typhoid Fever is a gastro-intestinal infection caused by ***Salmonella enterica typhi*** bacteria. It is transmitted from person to person – humans being the only reservoir – via the fecal-oral route where an infected or asymptomatic individual (does not exhibit symptoms) with poor hand or body hygiene passes the infection to another person when handling food and water. The bacteria multiply in the intestinal tract and can spread to the bloodstream. Paratyphoid fever, a similar illness, is caused by **Salmonella enterica paratyphi A, B, and C**.

Risk

The infection is endemic in many Southeast Asian countries as well as in Africa, Central and South America, and Western Pacific countries in areas where there is poor water and sewage sanitation. Floods in these regions can also quickly spread the bacteria. All travellers going to endemic areas are at risk, especially long term travellers, adventure travellers, humanitarian workers, and those visiting friends or relatives in areas of poor sanitation. Note that original infection does not provide immunity to subsequent infections.

Symptoms

Usually appear 1 to 3 weeks after exposure. Depending on the virulence of the infection symptoms can range from mild to severe. The illness is characterized by extreme fatigue and increasing fever. Other symptoms include headache, lack of appetite, malaise, and an enlarged liver. Sometimes patients have diarrhea, constipation, or a rash on their trunk. Severe symptoms may appear 2 to 3 weeks after onset illness and may include intestinal hemorrhage or perforation. Some people who recover from Typhoid or Paratyphoid Fever continue to be carriers of the bacteria and can potentially infect others. Treatment includes antibiotics and supportive care of symptoms. Unfortunately, **S. typhii** resistance to antibiotics is increasing worldwide.

Prevention

Wash your hands frequently and thoroughly, and practice proper body hygiene. Drink purified water (boiled or untampered bottled water) and only eat well cooked foods. Use the mantra **Boil it, Cook it, Peel it, or Forget it!**

Vaccination

There are two types of vaccines available; the inactivated injectable vaccine (lasting 2-3 years) and the live attenuated oral vaccine (lasting 5-7 years). Discuss your best options with your healthcare provider, including revaccination recommendations which differ in the USA and Canada. A combined Hepatitis A and Typhoid Fever vaccine is also available in Canada and Europe. Although typhoid vaccines do not provide 100% protection, they will reduce the severity of the illness. There is no vaccine available against Paratyphoid Fever.

Rabies

Description

Rabies is a viral infection caused by viruses belonging to the **Lyssavirus** genus. It is a zoonosis (an animal disease that can spread to humans) transmitted through the saliva of infected mammals bites. The infection primarily circulates among domestic and wild animals such as dogs, cats, monkeys, foxes, bats, raccoons, and skunks, although all mammals are at risk. The virus attacks the Central Nervous System targeting the brain and the spinal cord, and if untreated is fatal.

Risk

Rabies is present on all continents except Antarctica. The majority of human infections occur in Asia and Africa. Travellers coming into close contact with domestic animals or wildlife on ecotourism trips, or those undertaking outdoor activities like cave exploring, camping, trekking, and visiting farms or rural areas are at higher risk. Rabies is also an occupational hazard for veterinarians and wildlife researchers. Children are especially vulnerable since they may not report scratches or bites. They should be cautioned not to pet dogs, cats, monkeys, or other mammals. Any animal bite or scratch must be washed repeatedly with copious amounts of soap and water. Seek medical attention immediately.

Symptoms

Usually appear 1 to 3 months, although they can appear as early as a few days after being infected. The illness is characterized by fever and pain or a tingling sensation at the wound site. As a result of inflammation to the brain and spinal cord, some patients present with anxiety, hyperactivity, convulsions, delirium, and have a fear of swallowing or drinking liquids, as well as a fear of moving air or drafts. In other patients, muscles become paralysed followed by a coma. Once symptoms are present, most patients die within 1 or 2 weeks.

Prevention

Avoid contact with feral animals or wildlife. Try to anticipate an animal's actions and always be careful not to make sudden moves or surprise them. If you've been bitten by a mammal, wash the wound repeatedly and thoroughly with soap and water, and irrigate with an antiseptic. Seek medical attention immediately.

Vaccination

A series of 3 pre-exposure rabies vaccination shots is advised for persons planning an extended stay or on working assignments in remote and rural areas, particularly in Africa, Asia, Central and South America. The pre-exposure series simplifies medical care if the person has been bitten by a rabid animal and gives you enough time to travel back from a remote area to seek medical attention. Although this provides adequate initial protection, you will require 2 additional post-exposure doses if you are exposed to rabies. The preferred vaccines for rabies pre-exposure vaccination and post-exposure therapy are HDCV (Human Diploid Cell Rabies Vaccine) and PCECV (Purified Chick Embryo Cell Vaccine). These two vaccines are interchangeable.

Be aware that if you are in a remote area and are offered daily rabies treatment injections lasting 14 to 21 days, it may be one of the older animal brain-derived vaccines. We recommend that you do not take them due to serious side effects.

Note: Travellers who have not received the pre-exposure series need 4 to 5 shots of the rabies vaccine (depending on your health status) <u>and</u> the Human Rabies Immune Globulin (HRIG) which is calculated as 20 IU (International Units) per kilo of body weight. The full dose of HRIG should be injected into and around the bite site and if there is any remaining, it is given intramuscularly in another part of the body away from the wound. In some countries purified Equine Rabies Immune Globulin (ERIG) is used for post-exposure therapy when HRIG is not available. Note that HRIG is in short supply worldwide and is often not available in rural and remote areas.

General Health Risks

Air Pollution

Among the cities reporting to the World Health Organization, the following have the highest levels of particulate matter contributing to poor air quality: Monterrey, Toluca, Mexico city, Puebla and Salamanca .

Description

Outdoor air pollution is a mix of chemicals, particulate matter, and biological materials that react with each other to form tiny hazardous particles. It contributes to breathing problems, chronic diseases, increased hospitalization, and premature mortality.

The concentration of particulate matter (PM) is a key air quality indicator since it is the most common air pollutant that affects short term and long term health. Two sizes of particulate matter are used to analyze air quality; fine particles with a diameter of less than 2.5 µm or PM2.5 and coarse particles with a diameter of less than 10 µm or PM10. PM2.5 particles are more concerning because their small size allows them to travel deeper into the cardiopulmonary system.

The World Health Organization's air quality guidelines recommend that the annual mean concentrations of PM2.5 should not exceed 10 µm/m3 and 20 µm/m3 for PM10.

Risk

Cities and rural areas worldwide are affected by air pollution. When planning a trip, consider health status, age, destination, length of trip and season to mitigate the effects of air pollution.

Symptoms

Short term symptoms resulting from exposure to air pollution include itchy eyes, nose and throat, wheezing, coughing, shortness of breath, chest pain, headaches, nausea, and upper respiratory infections (bronchitis and pneumonia). It also exacerbates asthma and emphysema. Long term effects include lung cancer, cardiovascular disease, chronic respiratory illness, and developing allergies. Air pollution is also associated with heart attacks and strokes.

Prevention

- Comply with air pollution advisories - ask around and observe what locals are doing and avoid strenuous activities.
- Travellers with asthma or chronic obstructive pulmonary disease (COPD) should carry an inhaler, antibiotic, or oral steroid - consult your doctor to see what is best for you.

- Older travellers with pre-existing conditions should get a physical exam that includes a stress and lung capacity test prior to departure.
- Newborns and young children should minimize exposure as much as possible or consider not travelling to areas with poor air quality.
- Ask your medical practitioner if a face mask is advisable for you.

Altitude Illness

Pico de Orizaba (5700m / 18700ft), Iztaccihuatl (5280m / 17332ft) and La Malinche (4450m / 14600ft) are high altitude volcano summits in Mexico that attract climbers.

Description

Altitude Illness occurs as a result of decreased oxygen pressure at high altitudes. The illness is divided into three syndromes recognized by a cluster of symptoms arising from rapid ascent to high altitudes, especially more than 2400m / 7874ft.

Risk

All non-acclimatized travellers, including children, are potentially at risk of developing altitude illness which depends on level of exertion, speed of ascent, altitude reached, humidity, oxygen, and air pressure levels, as well as personal susceptibility. The human body is able to acclimatize to high altitude but must be given time to do so, ideally 3 to 5 days.

Symptoms

The first syndrome, Acute Mountain Sickness (AMS), is characterized by headache, fatigue, loss of appetite, nausea and sometimes vomiting, dizziness, insomnia and disturbed sleep appearing 2 to 12 hours after arrival at high altitude. Symptoms usually disappear within 24 to 72 hours as the body acclimatizes to the altitude. If AMS symptoms persist, rest and medication is needed. Do <u>not</u> continue to ascend to a higher altitude if symptoms persist. If there is no improvement descend to a lower altitude, by at least 300m / 984ft.

In rare cases AMS progresses to the second syndrome, High Altitude Cerebral Edema (HACE), which is characterized by worsening AMS symptoms, drowsiness, confusion, staggering gate and ataxia (lack of voluntary muscle coordination). Immediate descent to lower altitude is important since developing HACE symptoms can be life threatening if untreated immediately. HACE is rare at altitudes below 3600m / 11811ft.

The third syndrome, High Altitude Pulmonary Edema (HAPE), affects the lungs and is characterized by increased breathlessness with exertion progressing to breathlessness during rest, a dry cough, chest tightness or congestion, rapid heart beat, general weakness, and blue / purple skin tissue coloration. Developing HAPE symptoms can be life threatening if untreated. Immediate descent to a lower altitude and administration of oxygen are imperative.

Descending immediately, combined with medication (and oxygen, if available), is the best treatment for severe AMS, HACE, or HAPE. Consider evacuation if necessary.

Acclimatizing to high altitudes:

- Your ascent schedule should include rest days and flexibility in case you need to slow down and adjust to the new altitude. A gradual ascent to high altitude, possibly over a few days, is ideal. If this is not possible, make sure to allow extra time to acclimatize: 1 day for every 1000m / 3280ft.
- Avoid strenuous exercise for the first two days and avoid all alcoholic beverages for the first few days.
- Set a reasonable pace, avoid over exertion, and keep hydrated. Do not overload yourself with extra gear. If you are camping at high altitudes, ensure that there is good ventilation when using camp stoves and heaters in confined spaces.
- Consult with your healthcare provider if taking acetazolamide (Diamox) or other medication to help with acclimatization is appropriate for you.
- Persons with chronic medical conditions such as angina, heart failure, pulmonary diseases, and diabetes should consult with a high altitude medicine specialist before going travelling to mountainous areas.

Prevention

Plan your ascent over several days to ensure proper acclimatization (at altitudes of more than 2400m / 7874ft, ascend at a rate of no more than 300m / 984ft per day). Learn about the symptoms before you go and heed the warnings when symptoms appear. Do not continue to higher altitude, especially to sleep, when symptoms appear even if you feel they are minor. Descend to a lower altitude (at least 300m / 984ft) if symptoms persist while resting at your current altitude.

Chagas Disease

Chagas Disease is transmitted by the Triatoma insect in rural and suburban areas of Mexico, Central America, South America, and the southern United States.

Risk is present in all rural areas. The highest incidence rates are reported from the states of Chiapas, Distrito Federal, Hidalgo, Guerrero, Jalisco, Morelos, Nayarit, Oaxaca, Puebla, Querétaro, Veracruz, Yucatán, and Zacatecas. Only sporadic cases are reported from the two northern states of Chihuahua and Coahuila. The blood supply is not screened appropriately. Main vectors: *Triatoma dimidiata* is present in all affected areas; *Rhodnius prolixus* is present also in Oaxaca and Chiapas.

Description

Chagas Disease, also known as American Trypanosomiasis, is a protozoan infection transmitted by the Triatoma insect (known as 'vinchuca' in Spanish or 'barbeiro' in Portuguese) which bites humans most commonly on the face at night. The Triatoma insect sheds feces containing the **Trypanosoma cruzi** protozoa at the site of the bite which are rubbed or crushed into the bite wound to alleviate itching. The parasite then enters the bloodstream and affects organ tissues, typically the heart and the intestines. The disease largely spreads with the rise of migration from rural areas to urban and suburban areas as well as increasing deforestation. Chagas Disease affects between 7 and 8 million people and is a Neglected Tropical Disease (NTD)*. Many countries affected by the disease have active health education and eradication programs.

Neglected Tropical Diseases are chronic infections that are typically endemic in low income countries. They prevent affected adults and children from going to school, working, or fully participating in community life, contributing to stigma and the cycle of poverty.

Risk

Travellers undertaking outdoor activities such as hiking, camping, and ecotourism in endemic countries in Central and South America are at higher risk. Triatoma insects are found in forest ecosystems and poorly built homes, including huts and cabins. Chagas Disease can also be acquired via unscreened blood products, transmitted from mother to child during pregnancy, or by eating contaminated food and drinking unpasteurized fruit juices.

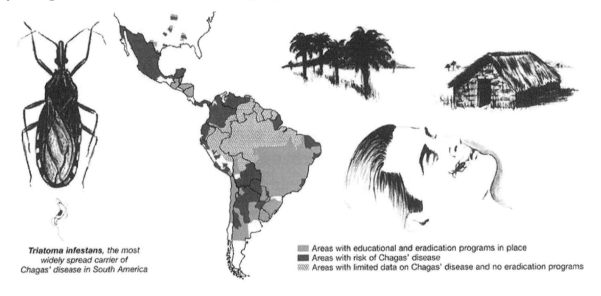

Triatoma infestans, the most widely spread carrier of Chagas' disease in South America

▓ Areas with educational and eradication programs in place
■ Areas with risk of Chagas' disease
░ Areas with limited data on Chagas' disease and no eradication programs

Symptoms

There are two phases of the illness. The majority of cases in the acute phase are asymptomatic (persons do not exhibit symptoms). For those that have symptoms, they usually appear 1 to 2 weeks after being infected and may include fever, swelling of the lymph nodes, enlarged liver, and in some cases swelling at the site of the bite usually on the face, hands, or feet. For most people, however, Chagas Disease is a silent infection showing up many years later often mimicking chronic heart conditions or as gastro-intestinal complications. Treatment includes taking anti-parasitic medications.

116

Prevention

One of the most effective ways to prevent Chagas Disease is to sleep under a permethrin-treated bed net. Also, avoid drinking unpasteurized juices and only eat well cooked foods or fruits that can be peeled. For complete information on prevention methods as well as transmission patterns and geographical distribution of Chagas Disease, see IAMAT's: Be Alert to Chagas Disease [59]

Chagas Disease Prevention Guidelines

- When travelling in endemic areas, do not sleep in huts since the *Triatoma* insects shelter in the palm-front roofs and in the wall cracks.
- When choosing a campsite, stay away from palm trees; do not set your tent close to stone or wood piles where the insects may be hiding.
- When checking into modest or older hotels (alojamientos), search for hidden insects under the mattress, behind picture frames, in drawers, or dark corners of the room. Carry insect and insecticides repellents with you.
- Before sleeping, apply insect repellent to exposed parts of your body (available in sprays, lotions, and towelettes), which may help to keep the insects away. Any commercially available preparation containing DEET (N, N-diethyl-meta-toluamide) is suitable.
- Use bed nets to prevent contact with insects. Put a cloth over the bed net to prevent the feces of infected insect from falling on you.
- Protect your hands with a cloth, paper, or gloves, if it is necessary to handle the insects.

Chikungunya

Mexico has confirmed Chikungunya cases. For the latest information on Chikungunya outbreaks please go to PAHO. [60]

Description

Chikungunya is a viral infection caused by the CHIK virus belonging to the Togaviridae family. The virus is transmitted through the bite of infected daytime biting female – primarily Aedes aegypti and Aedes albopictus – mosquitoes. They usually bite during the early morning and late afternoon, and are typically found in and around urban and suburban dwellings. Some mosquitoes that transmit Chikungunya in Africa also live in forested areas. Monkeys and other wild animals are also believed to be reservoirs or carriers of the virus.

Risk

Travellers going to the Caribbean, Central America, South America, sub-Saharan Africa, southeast Asia, and the Indian subcontinent are at risk, especially during the rainy season. Isolated cases of locally acquired Chikungunya have occurred in the USA, Italy and France.

Symptoms

In some cases, Chikungunya is asymptomatic – persons do not exhibit symptoms. Those with symptoms usually get ill 3-12 days after being bitten by an infected mosquito. Symptoms include sudden fever and severe muscle and joint pain. They can be accompanied by headache, fatigue nausea, vomiting, and a rash. Although most patients fully recover, chronic joint pain may last for several weeks or months. Other persistent problems may include eye, gastrointestinal, neurological, and heart complications. Persons with chronic health conditions, a weakened immune system, infants, and older persons are at risk of developing complications with this infection. Chikungunya is rarely fatal. Treatment includes supportive care of symptoms. There is no antiviral treatment available.

If you have had Chikungunya in the past, you are immune to subsequent infections. Chikungunya virus can be misdiagnosed for Zika Virus[61] or Dengue.[62]

Prevention

Travellers should take meticulous measures to prevent mosquito bites during the daytime.

- Use a repellent containing 20%-30% DEET or 20% Picaridin. Re-apply according to manufacturer's directions.
- Wear neutral-coloured (beige, light grey) clothing. If possible, wear long-sleeved, light-weight garments.
- If available, apply a permethrin spray or solution to clothing and gear.
- Get rid of water containers around dwellings and ensure that door and window screens work properly.
- Apply sunscreen first followed by the repellent (preferably 20 mintues later).
- More details on insect bite prevention.[63]

There is no preventive medication or vaccine against Chikungunya.

Dengue

The risk of Dengue is currently greatest along both the Pacific and Atlantic coastal areas, including the lower half of Baja California. The high altitude areas of central Mexico currently have no risk. Increased risk may occur during the rainy season, from July through October.

Mexico has confirmed Dengue cases nationally. *For the latest information on Dengue outbreaks please go to:* PAHO. [64]

Description

Dengue is a viral infection caused by four types of viruses (DENV-1, DENV-2, DENV-3, DENV-4) belonging to the *Flavivirdae* family. The viruses are transmitted through the bite of infected *Aedes aegypti* and *Aedes albopictu*s female mosquitoes that feed both indoors and outdoors during the daytime (from dawn to dusk). These mosquitoes thrive in areas with standing water, including puddles, water tanks, containers and old tires. Lack of reliable sanitation and regular garbage collection also contribute to the spread of the mosquitoes.

Risk

Risk of Dengue exists in tropical and subtropical areas of Central America, South America, Africa, Asia, and Oceania. All travellers are at risk during outbreaks. Long-term travellers and humanitarian workers going to areas where Dengue is endemic are at higher risk. Dengue occurs in urban and suburban settings with higher transmission rates happening during the rainy season.

Symptoms

In some cases, Dengue infection is asymptomatic – persons do not exhibit symptoms. Those with symptoms get ill between 4 to 7 days after the bite. The infection is characterized by flu-like symptoms which include a sudden high fever coming in separate waves, pain behind the eyes, muscle, joint, and bone pain, severe headache, and a skin rash with red spots. Treatment includes supportive care of symptoms. There is no antiviral treatment available.

The illness may progress to Dengue Hemorrhagic Fever (DHF). Symptoms include severe abdominal pain, vomiting, diarrhea, convulsions, bruising, and uncontrolled bleeding. High fever can last from 2 to 7 days. Complications can lead to circulatory system failure and shock, and can be fatal (also known as Dengue Shock Syndrome).

If you are infected with the same Dengue virus serotype you become immune to future infections. However, if you are infected subsequently with a different serotype, immunity wanes over time which increases the risk of developing Dengue Hemorrhagic Fever.

Dengue is related to Zika Virus,[65] Yellow Fever,[66] West Nile Virus,[67] and Japanese Encephalitis.[68] It can be misdiagnosed for Chikungunya,[69] Zika Virus,[70] or Yellow Fever.[71]

Prevention

Travellers should take meticulous measures to prevent mosquito bites during the daytime.

- Use a repellent containing 20%-30% DEET or 20% Picaridin. Re-apply according to manufacturer's directions.
- Wear neutral-coloured (beige, light grey) clothing. If possible, wear long-sleeved, light-weight garments.
- If available, apply a permethrin spray or solution to clothing and gear.
- Get rid of water containers around dwellings and ensure that door and window screens work properly.
- Apply sunscreen first followed by the repellent (preferably 20 mintues later.)
- More details on insect bite prevention. [72]

A vaccine is available for people living in some Dengue endemic countries, but is not commercially available for travellers.

Author's Note:

> According to recent information about the Mexican vaccine: Mexican authorities have declared that the vaccine is 60.5% effective against dengue, and 93.2% effective against severe dengue. This solution could help endemic countries bring down dengue deaths greatly. According to the Mexican government, this vaccine can help prevent more than 8,000 hospitalizations, over 100 deaths, and save the country 1.1 billion pesos in medical attention.
>
> Mexico reported 32,100 cases of dengue in 2014, and more than 8,000 were severe. In medical costs and equipment, the authorities reported over 3.2 billion Mexican pesos in expenses, which is about $187 million. However, Mexico isn't the only country developing a vaccine against the pesky disease. India has stepped up to the plate as well, but its vaccine is still at the animal trial stage. Knowing how reliable Indian medicine is, it's possible it's even better than the French-Mexican alternative.

Hepatitis E

Hepatitis E is highly endemic in Mexico.

Description

Hepatitis E (HEV) is a viral infection causing inflammation of the liver. It is primarily acquired by ingesting water contaminated with fecal matter. The virus is also transmitted from person to person through the fecal-oral route as a result of poor body hygiene practices. In some regions (Europe and Japan) pigs, deer, and wild boars are known to be reservoirs for the infection and Hepatitis E can be contracted by eating raw or undercooked meat such as pig liver and venison.

Risk

The infection is present worldwide, although its prevalence varies in different regions. Travellers drinking untreated water, eating undercooked meats, or going to areas with poor sanitation are at greater risk of Hepatitis E. The infection is present worldwide, although its prevalence varies in different regions.

Symptoms

Usually appear between 2 to 9 weeks after infection and include fever, fatigue, lack of appetite, abdominal pain, and jaundice. Treatment is based on alleviating the symptoms until they disappear.

Prevention

Only drink filtered or water treated with chlorine or iodine. Eat well cooked meats, and wash your hands frequently and thoroughly. There is currently no commercially available preventive vaccine or medication against Hepatitis E.

Cutaneous Larva Migrans

Description

Hookworm, also known as Cutaneous Larva Migrans (CLM), is a skin infection primarily caused by *Ancyclostoma braziliense* hookworms. It is acquired by walking barefoot or sitting on soil or sand contaminated with dog or cat feces containing hookworm larvae. The hookworm eggs hatch in the soil or sand and the larvae migrate through a person's skin forming red burrows or tracks underneath the outer skin layer.

Risk

Cutaneous Larva Migrans is prevalent in tropical and subtropical areas of the Caribbean, South America, Asia, and Africa, but can also occur during the hot months in temperate regions. Travellers taking beach vacations are at greater risk.

Symptoms

Usually symptoms include itching (which can cause a secondary bacterial infection), mild swelling, and redness at the place of larval penetration, typically on a person's feet or buttocks. The burrows or tracks usually appear 1 to 5 days after exposure, but sometimes can take weeks to show up. In the majority of cases the infection suddenly disappears after a few weeks. Treatment includes applying anti-itch creams and taking anthelmintic drugs.

Prevention

- Always wear shoes or sandals.
- At the beach, always sit on a towel and wash it after each use.
- Wash your hands and feet with soap and water, or if not available, use an alcohol-based hand sanitizer after touching sand or soil.

There is no preventive vaccine or medication against Hookworm.

Leishmaniasis

Cutaneous leishmaniasis is endemic in rural areas in the southern territory of Quintana Roo, eastern Yucatan, Campeche, eastern Tabasco, Chiapas, Oaxaca, and eastern Veracruz. Mucocutaneous leishmaniasis has occurred in Jalisco State, and visceral leishmaniasis has occurred in Guerrero and Morelos States. Cutaneous leishmaniasis occurs across both the northeast and southeast regions.

Description

Leishmaniasis is a parasitic infection caused by different species of *Leishmania* protozoa. It is transmitted through the bite of infected female sandflies belonging to the *Phlebotomus, Lutzomyia,* and *Psychodopygus* species. These nocturnal insects bite from dusk to dawn and are often found in forests, stone and mud walls cracks, and animal burrows. They are very tiny silent flyers – they do not hum – and their bite might go unnoticed. Leishmaniasis is clinically divided into three major categories – cutaneous, mucocutaneous, and visceral – and is a Neglected Tropical Disease (NTD)*.

*** Neglected Tropical Diseases are chronic infections that are typically endemic in low income countries. They prevent affected adults and children from going to school, working, or fully participating in community life, contributing to stigma and the cycle of poverty.**

Risk

Adventure travellers, bird watchers, missionaries, army personnel, construction workers, and researchers on night time assignments are at higher risk of being exposed to sand flies. **Cutaneous Leishmaniasis** is the most common form of the infection and is found in two geographic areas:

- Old World Cutaneous Leishmaniasis is present in the Mediterranean basin (southern Europe and North Africa), the Middle East, southwest and central Asia, and the tropical areas of Africa. The majority of cases are reported from the following countries: Afghanistan, Algeria, Iran, Iraq, Saudi Arabia and Syria. Old World cutaneous leishmaniasis is a mostly self-limiting skin disease in adults, but depending on the species, infected infants and children can develop the visceral form of the disease.

- New World Cutaneous Leishmaniasis is common in rural areas but can also be acquired in semi-urban and urban areas. It also occurs in rainforests and arid areas. New World cutaneous leishmaniasis is present in parts of North America (occasional cases are reported from the states of Texas and Oklahoma), Mexico, Central and South America, with Brazil and Peru reporting the majority of cases.

Symptoms of Cutaneous Leishmaniasis: Initial symptoms include skin lesions, which develop after several weeks or months after being infected, and swollen glands. The lesions - closed or open sores - can change overtime in size and appearance, they are usually painless, but can become painful if infected with bacteria. The lesions can take a long time to heal and usually leave scarring. Infections with some strains of New World cutaneous leishmaniasis may develop into **Mucocutaneous Leishmaniasis** years after the initial skin lesions seem to have healed completely. The infection spreads to the nose, mouth, and throat causing sores and bleeding. This complication can occur when the initial cutaneous leishmaniasis has not been treated.

Visceral Leishmaniasis, also know as kala-azar, is caused by some *Leishmania* species that invade the liver, spleen, bone marrow, and skin.

Symptoms of Visceral Leishmaniasis: Usually appear weeks or months after being infected and include fever, weight loss, and enlarged liver. Advanced untreated visceral leishmaniasis can be fatal, particularly if other underlying medical conditions such as tuberculosis, pneumonia, and dysentry are present. This form of Leishmaniasis is very rare in travellers but it affects local populations in remote areas of India, Nepal, Bangladesh, Sudan, South Sudan, Ethiopia, and Brazil.

Prevention

Avoid dusk to dawn outdoor activities. Presoak protective clothing with permethrin insecticide. Use insect repellent containing DEET on exposed skin and sleep under permethrin treated bed nets or in air conditioned areas. (Sand flies are very small, 2-3 mm, and may be able to enter through regular screens and nettings. Insecticide treated screens and nets can reduce risk of entry). There is no preventive vaccination or medication against leishmaniasis. Treatment options depend on identifying the infective *leishmania* species and the extent of the infection, but generally includes antifungal and antibacterial ointments.

Malaria

Malaria is transmitted by the night-time - dusk to dawn - biting female Anopheles mosquito.

Malaria - Overview How to Protect Yourself Against Malaria [73]

World Malaria Risk Chart [74]

Risk is present in the country; areas of risk are specified:

- Pacific Coast: areas of Sonora, Chihuahua, Sinaloa, Durango, Nayarit, and Jalisco. Take meticulous anti-mosquito bite measures from dusk to dawn when travelling in rural areas of these states.
- Southern Mexico: Rural areas of Chiapas and Oaxaca, sporadic cases are also reported from rural areas of Tabasco, Campeche and Quintana Roo (the forested areas bordering Belize and Guatemala). Take any one of the antimalarial medications listed below for these areas.
- Archaeological sites: Daytime excursions from cities to popular archeological sites do not require antimalarial medication. However, travellers staying overnight in the vicinity or in nearby villages of the following sites should take one of the antimalarial medications listed below.
- Chiapas (Bonampak, El Cayo, La Mar, Palenque, Toniná, etc.). Cities of Villahermosa and Tuxtla Gutierrez are risk free.
- Campeche (Becan, Calakmul, Edzná, Hochob, Xpuhil, etc.). City of Campeche is risk free.

Note: Travellers to rural areas and major resorts along both coasts (Acapulco, Puerto Vallarta, etc.) should take meticulous anti-mosquito bite measures from dusk to dawn.

Malaria risk is present below the altitude of: 1000 meters

Malaria transmission vector(s): *A.albimanus*

Incidence of *Plasmodium falciparum* Malaria: 0% Of the five species of human malaria parasites, *Plasmodium falciparum* is the most dangerous. The remaining percentage represents malaria infections that may be caused by one or more of the following parasites: *Plasmodium vivax, Plasmodium ovale, Plasmodium malariae, and Plasmodium knowlesi.*

Suppressive Medication Guide

All malaria infections are serious illnesses and must be treated as a medical emergency. In offering guidance on the choice of antimalarial drugs, the main concern is to provide protection against *Plasmodium falciparum* malaria, the most dangerous and often fatal form of the illness.

Regardless of the medication which has been taken, it is of utmost importance for travellers and their physician to consider fever and flu-like symptoms appearing 7 days up to several months after leaving a malarious area as a malaria breakthrough. Early diagnosis is essential for successful treatment.

In addition to the suggested antimalarial medication, use a mosquito bed net and effective repellents to avoid the bite of the nocturnal *Anopheles* mosquito.

Did you know that Malaria is preventable?

The **How to Protect Yourself Against Malaria** whitepaper discusses the life cycle of the Malaria parasite and offers mechanical and pharmaceutical protection guidelines. It also details medication dosages, side-effects, and contraindications, as well as alternative protection measures for pregnant travellers, children, and people with special needs and drug sensitivities.

The medications listed below are effective against malaria in this country. Discuss with your healthcare provider which antimalarial regimen is best suited to your needs. Take ONE of the following:

Chloroquine

- Take in weekly doses of 500 mg (300 mg base).
- Start 1 week before entering malarious area, continue weekly during your stay and continue for 4 weeks after leaving. Take it after a meal to avoid stomach upsets.
- **Note:** The bitter taste makes the drug unpalatable. Minor stomach upsets, itching skin, nausea and diarrhea may occur. It may also cause blurred vision and a transitory headache.

Hydrochloroquine

- Take in weekly doses of 400 mg (310 mg base).
- Start 1 week before entering malarious area, continue weekly during your stay and continue for 4 weeks after leaving.
- **Note:** An alternative to chloroquine that may be better tolerated.

Atovaquone-proguanil

- Brand names: *Malarone, Malanil* and others; generics available.
- Take 1 tablet daily (atovaquone 250 mg + Proguanil 100 mg).

- Start 1-2 days before entering the malarious area, continue daily during your stay and continue fore 7 days after leaving.
- **Note:** Take at the same time every day with food or milk.

Doxycycline

- Brand names: *Vibramycin* and others; generics available.
- Take 1 tablet daily (100 mg).
- Start 1 day before entering malarious area, continue daily during your stay and continue for 4 weeks after leaving.
- **Note:** When taking this drug, avoid exposure to direct sunlight and use sunscreen with protection against long range ultraviolet radiation (UVA) to minimize risk of photosensitive reaction. Take with large amounts of water to prevent esophageal and stomach irritation.

Mefloquine hydrochloride

- Brand names: *Lariam, Mephaquin, Mefliam* and others; generics available.
- Take 1 tablet of 250 mg (228 mg base) once a week.
- Start 1-2 weeks before entering the malarious area, continue weekly during your stay and continue fore 4 weeks after leaving.
- **Note:** Side effects include nausea and headache, including neurological side effects such as dizziness, ringing of the ears, and loss of balance. Psychiatric side effects include anxiety, depression, mistrustfulness, and hallucinations. Neurological side effects can occur any time during use and can last for long periods of time or become permanent even after the drug is stopped. Seek medical advice if any neurological or psychiatric side effects occur.

For further details, cautions, contraindications, or alternatives, including guidelines for pediatric dosages and Emergency Self Treatment, download our whitepaper How to Protect Yourself Against Malaria.[75]

The recommendations for malaria prophylaxis outlined here are intended as guidelines only and may differ according to where you live, your health status, age, destination, trip itinerary, type of travel, and length of stay. Seek further advice from your physician or travel health clinic for the malaria prophylactic regimen most appropriate to your needs.

Sexually Transmitted Infections

Description

Sexually transmitted infections (STIs), also known as Sexually Transmitted Diseases (STDs), are caused by bacteria, viruses or parasites and are transmitted via unprotected sex (vaginal, anal, or oral) and skin to skin genital contact.

Bacterial infections include Bacterial Vaginosis, Chlamydia, Gonorrhea, Lyphogranuloma venerum (LGV) and Syphilis. Viruses cause Genital Herpes, Hepatitis B, Human Papillomavirus (HPV) and Human Immunodeficiency Virus (HIV). Parasites are responsible for Trichomoniasis and pubic lice.

STIs occur worldwide, but some infections like chancroid, lymphogranuloma vernerum (LGV), and Granuloma Inguinale are more common in less industrialized countries.

Zika Virus [76] can also be sexually transmitted through infected semen. More research is needed, but men who have shown symptoms of Zika Virus can transmit the infection to their partners. Scientists still do not know if an infected man who does not develop symptoms can sexually transmit the virus. So far, there have been no cases of infected women sexually transmitting the virus.

Risk

Travellers are at high risk of acquiring STIs if they have unprotected sex outside a monogamous relationship, engage in casual sex, or use the services of sex workers. During travel, some people may be less inclined to follow social mores dictating their behaviour back home and look for adventurous opportunities involving sex. Long term travellers may also be at increased risk due to feelings of loneliness or being homesick.

Travellers should also be aware of sexual tourism and how it spreads STIs. Sexual tourism is travel for the procurement of sex abroad. Travellers participating in this type of exploitive tourism use the services of sex workers or children that are forced to engage in the trade as a result of deceptive practices or are part of human trafficking networks. It's illegal in many countries and you can be prosecuted in your home country for engaging in sexual exploitation of minors abroad. Sexual violence such as rape or assault can also increase risk of STI.

Symptoms

In many cases you can spread a sexually transmitted infection unknowingly because you are asymptomatic (do not exhibit symptoms). Depending on the infection, symptoms can appear within days or weeks (Chlamydia, Gonorrhea, Genital Herpes), weeks or months (Hepatitis B, Syphilis, HIV) after the initial infection. Common symptoms, which may appear alone or in combination include abnormal genital discharge, burning sensation when urinating, bleeding after intercourse or between periods, rashes and sores in the genital or anal areas, swollen lymph glands in the groin, and sudden fever or appearance of flu-like symptoms.

Note that the sudden or eventual disappearance of symptoms does not mean you are cured from the infection since it can return or manifest itself in different symptoms. Many sexually transmitted infections can be treated with antibiotics (although there is mounting evidence that Gonorrhea is becoming increasingly resistant to antibiotics) or antivirals. If left untreated, infections can lead to infertility, pelvic inflammatory disease, cancer, chronic liver conditions, pregnancy complications, and birth defects.

Prevention

Always practice safe sex. Pack your own male and / or female condoms. Note that condoms obtained abroad may have higher breakage rates, may be expired, or may have been stored in hot or humid places compromising their effectiveness. Use your condom correctly and do not use oil based lubes. If you engage in oral sex use a male condom or dental dam. Keep in mind that birth control methods such as oral contraceptives, injections, IUDs, or diaphragms do not prevent STI transmission, and that condoms aren't fully effective from infections acquired via skin-to-skin contact like genital herpes.

Avoid behaviour that increases your chances of contracting an STI such as casual sex with a stranger or a sex worker. Drinking heavily or taking mind-altering drugs will impair your judgement and inhibitions during a sexual encounter, putting you at risk of making unsafe choices like not using a condom. If you already practice safe sex, avoid getting tattoos, body piercings, or acupuncture treatments. Also don't share razors, toothbrushes, or needles. If you have engaged in risky sexual activities or suspect that you may have an STI, visit a healthcare provider immediately. If the results confirm that you have an STI, inform all your sex partners and encourage them to seek medical attention.

Hepatitis B[77] and Human Papillomavirus (HPV) can also be prevented through vaccination.

Note: Some countries continue to have entry restrictions for travellers with HIV / AIDS. Consult your destination country's embassy or consulate to get the latest information. See also HIVTravel [78] for details.

Soil-Transmitted Helminths

Highly prevalent in most rural areas.

Description

Parasitic worms are organisms that can live and replicate in the gastro-intestinal system. These soil-transmitted helminths (hookworms, roundworms, whipworms) are transmitted through the fecal-oral route as a result of poor sanitary practices. The most common infections that can affect travellers are Ascariasis, Hookworm, and Trichuriasis which are Neglected Tropical Diseases (NTDs)*.

* Neglected Tropical Diseases are chronic infections that are typically endemic in low income countries. They prevent affected adults and children from going to school, working, or fully participating in community life, contributing to stigma and the cycle of poverty.

Risk

Travellers can get ill when worm eggs are ingested by:

- Eating raw, unwashed, or improperly handled fruits and vegetables.
- Drinking contaminated water or beverages.
- Touching the mouth with dirty hands or through improper hand washing.

- Practising poor body hygiene.

Ascariasis: The infection is caused by *Ascaris lumbricoides* roundworm and is typically found in tropical and sub-tropical areas. Persons with light infections may not exhibit any symptoms. Those who develop symptoms start with a persistent cough, wheezing, shortness within 1 week of getting infected as a result of larvae migrating to the lungs and throat. The second set of symptoms, including abdominal pain, nausea, vomiting, diarrhea, bloody or worm in stools, fatigue, weight loss appear a few weeks (up to 2 or 3 months) later as the roundworms become adults and the females lay eggs which are shed through feces. The parasite can live in humans for up to 2 years. Children are particularly affected by this illness because they tend to play in and eat dirt. Treatment includes taking anthelmintic drugs.

Hookworm | Ancyclostomiasis: This intestinal infection is primarily caused by *Necator americanus*, followed by *Ancylostoma duodenale*, and to a lesser extent by *Ancylostoma ceylanicum* nematodes typically found in tropical and sub-tropical areas. Persons with light infections may not exhibit any symptoms. Those who develop symptoms first get a skin rash where the larvae penetrate the skin. Abdominal pain, diarrhea, loss of appetite, weight loss, and fatigue occur as the migrated larvae grow into adults and mate in the gastro-intestinal system. The eggs produced by the females are shed through feces. Note that the *Ancylostoma duodenale* hookworm can also be acquired by ingesting soil or sand through dirty hands or unwashed fruits and vegetables. A typical sign of this infection is anemia (iron deficiency). Treatment includes taking anthelmintic drugs.

Trichuriasis: The infection in humans is caused by the *Trichuris trichuria* whipworm and occurs worldwide, especially in areas with no proper sewage disposal. Persons with light infections may not exhibit any symptoms. Those who exhibit symptoms have diarrhea, containing blood, mucous, and water as a result of the swallowed eggs hatching in the caecum, the pouch-like area of the large intestine, and the larvae migrate to the lining the colon to grow into adulthood and mate. The eggs produced by the females are shed through feces. Severe cases include abdominal pain, chronic diarrhea, and rectal prolapse. Whipworms can live in humans for years. Children are particularly affected by this illness because they tend to play in and eat dirt. Treatment includes taking anthelmintic drugs.

Traveller's Diarrhea

Description

The term Traveller's Diarrhea is used to describe gastro-intestinal infections affecting travellers caused by ingesting bacteria, viruses, and protozoa. These micro-organisms are found worldwide and are typically transmitted from person to person via the fecal-oral route – an infected person who does not practice proper hand or body hygiene passes on the infection to another person when handling food and water. Traveller's Diarrhea is the most common illness among travellers.

Risk

Traveller's Diarrhea can happen when:

- Eating raw, under cooked, unwashed, or improperly handled meat, poultry products, dairy products, fruits, vegetables, shellfish, and seafood.
- Drinking contaminated water or beverages.
- Inadvertently ingesting fecal matter, protozoa eggs, or viruses by touching the mouth with dirty or improperly washed hands.
- Eating out in restaurants, from buffets, or from street vendors where food handling and hygienic practices are not followed properly.

Prevention

The golden rule to prevent gastro-intestinal infections is: **Boil it, Cook it, Peel it, or Forget it!** However, it's not just about <u>what</u> you eat, it's also important to consider <u>where</u> you eat. It's not always easy to know if a restaurant or food vendor follows proper food handling and hygienic practices (properly cleaning cutting boards, utensils, sink to wash hands, refrigeration). Be cautious of food that has been stored uncovered, has been improperly refrigerated, or has been standing out for a long time such as buffets.

Consult your doctor for the best treatment options tailored to your needs, including taking prescription medication on your trip in case you suffer from diarrhea. Travellers with chronic conditions are more susceptible to infections and should consider taking preventive medication.

Get helpful reminders on food and water safety basics, including tips on what to do if you get sick. For more information on food and water safety download the following Tip Sheets from our eLibrary: How To Prevent Traveller's Diarrhea [79]

Did you know that Traveller's Diarrhea is the most common travel-related illness? Sometimes it's easy to forget or ignore health considerations that we take for granted back home. Fortunately, gastrointestinal infections can be prevented by being discerning about your food and water.

Food contamination due to *E. coli*, *salmonella*, or *listeria* can occur anywhere in the world, including at home. However, when you travel, you need to be more aware of where your food comes from.

Get quick tips on how to prevent food and water illnesses during your trip.

How To Prevent Food and Water Illnesses [80]

Did you know that washing your hands prevents many travel-related illnesses? Following good hand hygiene is not only good for your health; your pocketbook will thank you for not having to make itinerary changes, pay re-booking fees and deal with unexpected medical costs due to illness abroad.

This Tip Sheet shows how to properly wash your hands (yes, most of us don't do a good job) and the reasons why good hand hygiene is so important, not only to your own health, but to those around you. How To Prevent Illness by Washing Your Hands [81]

Zika Virus

There is a current outbreak of Zika virus in Mexico. States confirming recent cases include: Jalisco, Michoacán, Chiapas, Oaxaca, Guerrero, Tabasco and Veracruz.

For the latest information on Zika virus outbreaks please go to: PAHO.[82]

Description

Zika Virus infection is caused by the Zika Virus (ZIKV) belonging to the ***Flaviviridae*** family. It is a zoonosis (an animal disease that can spread to humans) primarily transmitted by infected daytime biting female ***Aedes aegypti*** and ***Aedes albopictus*** mosquitoes which are typically active from dawn to dusk. There is evidence that Zika Virus is also transmitted by other mosquitoes belonging to the ***Aedes*** genus.

Risk

Zika Virus is present in Mexico, Central America, South America, the Caribbean, tropical areas of Southeast Asia, Oceania, and parts of Africa. All travellers are at risk. Long-term travellers and aid or missionary workers going to areas where Zika Virus is endemic are at greater risk.

Information about the virus is continuously evolving. However, there is strong scientific consensus that Zika Virus causes neurological complications: Guillain-Barré syndrome (progressive muscle weakness that can lead to temporary paralysis) and microcephaly (decreased head size which may lead to developmental delays) in infants born to pregnant women infected with the virus.

The virus can be sexually transmitted through semen by men who reported having symptoms. However, it's still not clear if a man who does not develop symptoms can sexually transmit the virus. There also have been no cases of women sexually transmitting the virus. In some patients, researchers have found that the virus can be shed through saliva and urine.

Symptoms

In the majority of cases, Zika Virus infection is asymptomatic (persons do not exhibit symptoms). Those with symptoms usually get ill 3-12 days after being bitten by an infected mosquito. Symptoms include mild fever, headache, muscle and joint pain, nausea, vomiting, and general malaise. The illness is characterized by pink eye (inflammation of the conjunctiva), a skin rash with red spots on the face, neck, trunk, and upper arms which can spread to the palms or soles, and sensitivity to light. Some may also have a lack of appetite, diarrhea, abdominal pain, constipation, and dizziness. Most people fully recover from the illness within 7 days. Treatment includes supportive care of symptoms. There is no antiviral treatment available.

The Zika Virus is related to Dengue,[83] Yellow Fever,[84] West Nile Virus,[85] and Japanese Encephalitis.[86] It may be misdiagnosed for Dengue[87] and Chikungunya.[88]

Prevention

Travellers who are pregnant or planning to get pregnant should postpone travel to areas with Zika Virus outbreaks. Those who plan to travel to areas with Zika Virus should take meticulous measures to prevent mosquito bites during the daytime. Insect-bite prevention measures include applying a DEET-containing repellent to exposed skin, applying permethrin spray (or solution) to clothing and gear, wearing long sleeves and pants, getting rid of water containers around dwellings and ensuring that door and window screens work properly. There is currently no preventive medication or vaccine against Zika Virus.

To reduce the risk of sexual transmission, practice safe sex - use a condom correctly and consistently or abstain from sex. Both men and women who plan to visit, are returning from, or have recently lived in a country where Zika Virus is active, should practice safe sex for 8 weeks. Men who develop Zika Virus symptoms should practice safe sex for at least 6 months.

Tuberculosis

Tuberculosis is highly endemic in Mexico, especially among the native Indian populations in southern Mexico and Baja California. Multidrug-resistant strains are common.

Description

Tuberculosis (TB) is an airbone bacterial infection caused by *Mycobacterium tuberculosis*. TB can be acquired by breathing contaminated air droplets coughed or sneezed by a person nearby who has active Tuberculosis. Humans can also get ill with TB by ingesting unpasteurized milk products contaminated with *Mycobacterium bovis*, also known as Bovine Tuberculosis. The most common form of the infection is pulmonary TB which affects the lungs. In some cases, the bacteria can also attack the lymphatic system, central nervous system, urogenital area, joints, and bones.

Risk

Tuberculosis occurs worldwide and commonly spreads in cramped, overcrowded conditions. There is no evidence that pulmonary TB is more easily transmitted in airplanes or other forms of public transportation. Travellers with a compromised immune system, long-term travellers, and those visiting friends and relatives (VFR travellers) in areas where Tuberculosis is endemic are at greater risk. Humanitarian and healthcare personnel working in communities with active TB are also at increased risk. Persons with active TB should not travel.

Symptoms

Persons with active TB have symptoms which include excessive coughing (sometimes with blood), chest pain, general weakness, lack of appetite, weight loss, swollen lymph glands, fever, chills, and night sweats. It can be misdiagnosed for bronchitis or pneumonia. If untreated, active TB can lead to fatalities.

The majority of persons with the illness (90% to 95%) have latent TB infection (LTBI) and do not exhibit any symptoms. The bacteria can remain inactive for many years and the chance of developing active TB diminishes over time.

Tuberculosis treatment involves taking antibiotics for a minimum of 6 months. Drug-resistant TB is a major concern as an increasing number of people are no longer able to be treated with previously effective drugs. Due to misuse of antibiotic therapies, patients can develop multi-drug resistant Tuberculosis (MDR TB). When a second line of antibiotics fail to cure the multi-drug resistant infection, it is known as extensively drug-resistant Tuberculosis (XDR TB).

Prevention

Avoid exposure to people known to who have active Tuberculosis and only consume pasteurized milk products. Travellers at higher risk should have a pre-departure tuberculin skin test (TST) and be re-tested upon their return home. Those at increased risk should also consult their healthcare provider to determine if the Bacillus Calmette-Guérin (BCG) vaccine is recommended.

Factors Affecting Mental Health During Travel

Travel is enjoyable, but there is no doubt that it can be stressful. Even if you don't have a prior history of mental illness, travel stress, mood changes, anxiety and other mental health concerns can unexpectedly affect you and potentially disrupt your trip. Studies show that psychiatric emergencies are the leading cause for air evacuations along with injuries and cardiovascular disease.

Your mental and physical health prior to, and during, a trip determines how well you will cope with travel stress. Consider the following:

- Tiredness, lack of sleep.
- Major life events occurring prior to travel such as a birth, death, wedding, divorce, moving, or serious illness.
- Difficult home or professional life; experiencing recent emotional exhaustion or financial strain.
- Being lonely; prone to depression and anxiety.
- Having pre-existing psychiatric, behavioural, neurological disorders; memory or cognitive deficits.
- Dependence on, or misuse, of psychoactive substances.
- Using medications that have psychiatric or neurological side effects (some anti-retrovirals and anti-malarials).
- Type and length of travel; adventure, business, leisure, emergency aid work, missions.
- Travel destination; travelling to politically unstable or war-torn areas, returning to a place where psychological trauma occurred.

Mental Health Abroad

Mental illness is an under recognized public health concern and travellers often have difficulty accessing adequate emergency psychiatric care abroad. While some countries are leading the way in mental healthcare and treatment, 41% don't have dedicated mental health legislation.

According to the World Health Organization Mental Health Atlas, accessibility to a psychiatrist varies from 0.05 per 100,000 in Africa to 8.59 per 100,000 in Europe. All countries except European ones have less than 2 beds per 100,000 people in psychiatric wards located in general hospitals.*

Persons with mental health concerns have the additional burden of dealing with stigma, negative attitudes and behaviour towards their illness. Prejudice and discrimination towards mental illness may determine the type of medical care you will receive abroad.

- Tips for coping with travel stress.[89]
- Tips for travellers with: Mood disorders (depression, bipolar disorder) [90]

- Tips for travellers with: Anxiety disorders (panic attacks, phobias, obsessive compulsive disorders, posttraumatic stress disorder) [91]
- Tips for travellers with: Psychotic disorders (acute situational psychosis, schizophrenia)[92]

[Editor's Note: this is the ending of the helpful and authoritative information from IAMAT. We thank them for their worldwide support of travelers (or travellers as they would spell it as they use British spellings throughout) and their contribution to those who read this book and visit Mexico. We encourage you to visit their website and become a member. Membership is free, although donations are appreciated.[93]]

The Language Gap

International Living's Global Retirement Index for 2017 just ranked Mexico the top retirement destination in the world. Among the many reasons for this distinction is that Mexico has ranked above most in the many of the health- and medicine-related factors it considers. This ranking considers both cost and quality of care, the number of people per doctor, the number of hospital beds per thousand people, the percentage of the population with access to safe water, infant mortality, life expectancy and public health expenditure as a percentage of a country's GDP.

Of course, it is one thing to know that affordable quality care is available, and quite another for an English speaker to access it. In a recent exchange of comments on a Mexperience.com healthcare article we discussed the "language gap." It boils down to this fundamental question: If you don't speak fluent Spanish, are you going to be able to get the medical attention you need? Even in an emergency?

If you are prepared for the realities and are armed with some pertinent information, the answer is "yes." But it isn't going to just happen automatically. You really need to think about this now, before the need arises. Here are some of the things you may want to consider:

Plan Ahead

If possible, find an English-speaking primary care physician before you need care. If you require a specialist on a regular basis, establish that relationship as soon as you can, too. Don't wait until there is a crisis to find a doctor. Get a referral to an English-speaking physician or consider the companion to this book available on Amazon.com and Mexperience.com. [*See Appendix A: The English Speaker's Guide to Doctors & Hospitals in Mexico*]. If you have a resident's visa and IMSS, get your physical as soon as possible so you will get assigned to a general practitioner. You may be fortunate enough to be assigned to someone who speaks English.

Learn Spanish

Spanish is the native language of Mexico. As a non-native English speaker, please don't feel that Mexicans have an obligation to know your language. Many do speak English, and it is a great blessing for English-speakers, but it's our responsibility to bridge the "language gap."

For travel in Mexico, learning at least the kinds of phrases that might prove life-saving—and those greetings and polite phrases that make it clear that you are a caring person and consider each individual you meet worthy of consideration. [*See Helpful & Potentially Lifesaving Language Tips*] If you are thinking about Mexico as a permanent full- or part-time home it will be essential to learn more Spanish for effective day-to-day communication and to avoid the trap of social isolation. We highly recommend that you start to study immediately.

In a day and age when people are encouraged to pursue expensive "brain exercise" programs to stave off mental deterioration, learning a new language—beginning at any age—is relatively inexpensive and more effective at forming new neuron pathways in your brain than the "games" that are sometimes encouraged. Retirement should not be the occasion to cease learning. If anything, it becomes more important to use your mind to maintain its flexibility and learning Spanish will give you back far more than you put into it, certainly better for that than endless rounds of cards, crosswords or Sudoku.

When you begin to incorporate a bit of study into your daily routine, you may find, as many do, that learning Spanish is a pleasure to and speaking Spanish makes life infinitely easier in a Spanish-speaking country. Even if you will be in town or city with a significant expat community, please learn some Spanish. Every bit you learn helps, and Mexicans will appreciate your efforts, even those that speak English. Mexicans are very polite people and you need to learn, at the bare minimum, how to greet and thank people to not be thought rude.

My favorite online Spanish course is with Rocket Languages.[94] You set your own pace and work toward accurate pronunciation using a microphone.

Practice Being a Patient Patient

Many medical professionals in Mexico have some level of English proficiency, but it's wise to be considerate of possible language limitations by speaking slowly and clearly. Use a simple vocabulary. It's rude to grow impatient with someone who is trying to help you. Don't expect everyone to speak English, and even those that do may not be fluent.

Keep a Glossary on Hand

Be prepared for those instances where you may need emergency treatment from medical professionals that don't speak English. How? Consider printing out and carrying an English/Spanish translation of common medical terms and phrases, symptoms, body parts, etc. [*See Helpful & Potentially Lifesaving Language Tips*]

Communication is essential for most relationships in life and your relationship with health care providers is no exception. If you are willing to do your best to plan ahead and bridge the language gap by learning some Spanish and knowing where to turn to find English-speaking professionals, the people of Mexico will reward you with some of the best care available in the world right now.

Helpful & Potentially Lifesaving Language Tips

Urgent! You Must Learn This!

The most important thing to learn in any language isn't, "Where's the bathroom?" It is how to YELL FOR HELP! You don't want to find yourself in an urgent situation and not know how to summon people to your aid. Just screaming isn't enough. You need to scream "¡Auxilio! ¡Auxilio!" (help me). The way you say it is OX ZEE YO! Learn it. Your life could depend on it.

Giving Directions

Giving someone like an ambulance service directions during an emergency can be highly stressful and this is compounded when you don't speak the language or don't know exactly where you are. Here are some tips. If you are using a cell phone, keep it turned on. Your GPS signal may help others locate you.

Street addresses are not always available or useful in Mexico. People are very accustomed to navigating by landmarks and distances. So unless an address is obvious, or there is someone near to ask, don't waste time trying to find an address in an emergency. Give landmarks instead.

I am near (landmark). Estoy cerca de   .

I am (direction) of (landmark). Estoy   de   .

> (north, norte) (south, sur) (east, este) (west, oeste)
>
> (to the right, a la derecha)
>
> (to the left, a la izquierda)

These can be useful landmarks:

- kilometer markings on a road (kilometer numero)
- nearest place (lugar) or town (pueblo)
- store names (tienda) or other building (edificio)
- nearby crossroad (cruzado de caminos) or exit (salida de camino)
- natural features like a river (rio) or mountains (montañas)
- man-made features like a bridge (puente), high tension wire (cable de alta tension), sign
  (signo) or billboard (espectacular)

Communicating in Spanish (for the English Speaker)

Although there are medical professionals in Mexico who are fully bilingual, you should not assume that anyone will be able to communicate with you in English when you seek medical help. It is your responsibility to bridge the gap, not the other way around. When you seek medical treatment for an illness or injury, it is essential that, at a minimum, you be prepared to describe what is going on in Spanish. This guide can help.

Remember, the Mexican people are typically generous and patient with foreigners. You can repay this kindness by making an effort to use Spanish, even if it is very minimal, and by being polite. Greeting people, saying "thank you" and saying goodbye are an essential part of every social encounter including visits to the doctor. People thank the bus driver in Mexico to give you an idea of how important good manners and appreciation are.

Remember, even if a person speaks English, it may be very basic, so keep it simple. Also, speaking Spanglish (mixing English and Spanish) is okay in an urgent situation. Talking like Tarzan in Spanish or English is okay too.

Here are some helpful Spanish phrases:

Hello. *Hola*

Thank you. *Gracias*

Yes. *Sí*

No. *No*

Do you speak English? *Habla ingles?*

I need help. *Necesito ayuda.*

Help me please! *Ayúdame por favor!*

I am very sick. *Estoy muy infermo.*

I have been injured. *Me lastimé.*

How much does this cost? *Cuánto cuesta? Can you please… Podrías…*

I can / cannot… *Yo puedo / no puedo…*

I need… *Yo necesito…*

Where is the… *Dónde está el/la…*

Please take me to the …. *Por favor lléveme al/ a la*

This is / These are my… *Este(a/o) es / Estas(os) son mis…*

Goodbye. *Adios*

See you later. *Hasta luego.*

Thank you for your help. *Gracias por su ayuda.*

Important Nouns

bathroom	baño
battery	batería
doctor	doctor / doctora (fem)
elevator	ascensor
entrance / exit	entrada / salida
medicine	medicina
oxygen	oxígeno
phone	teléfono
ramp	rampa
wheelchair	silla de ruedas

Key Verbs

climb	escalar
close	cerrar
fall	caerse
find	encontrar
hear	escuchar
move	mover

Body Parts

allergy	alergia
ankle	el tobillo
arm	el brazo
back	la espalda
bladder	la vejiga
bleeding	dolor
blister	amolla
blood	la sangre
body	el cuerpo

bone	el hueso
bone	hueso
brain	el cerebro
breast	la mama
breathing	respiración
broken	fracturado
burn	quemar
calf	la pantorrilla
cartilage	cartílago
cheek	la mejilla
chest	el pecho
chills	escalofríos
chin	la barbilla
chocking	calce
constipation	estreñimiento
coughing	tos
cramps	calambres
depressed	deprimido
diarrhea	diarrea
dimple	el hoyuelo
dizzy	mareado
ear	la oreja
elbow	el codo
emergency	emergencia
eye	el ojo
eyebrow	la ceja
eyelashes	las pestañas
eyelid	el párpado
face	la cara
faint/lightheaded	desmayar/voy desmayar
fear	miedo

fever	fiebre
finger	el dedo
fist	el puño
foot/feet	el pie/s
forehead	la frente
freckle	la peca
hair	el pelo
hand	la mano
head	la cabeza
heart	el corazón
high blood pressure	hipertensión
hip	la cadera
infected	infectado
itching	picazón
jaw	la mandíbula
kidney	el riñón
knee	la rodilla
leg	la pierna
liver	el hígado
lump	bulto
lung	el pulmón
medication	medicación
mouth	la boca
muscle	el músculo
neck	el cuello
nipple	el pezón
nose	la nariz
open	abrir
pain	dolor
penis	el pene
puncture	punción

reach	alcanzar
rectum	el recto
see	ver
seizure	incautación
shoulder	el hombro
skin	la piel
smell	olor
sore	llaga
sting	aguijón
stomach	el estómago
swollen	hinchado
talk	hablar
testicle	el testículo
thigh	el muslo
throat	la garganta
throbbing	palpitante
thumb	el pulgar
tongue	la lengua
tooth	el diente
twisted	retorcido
urine	orina
vagina	la vagina
vein	la vena
vomiting	vómitos
waist	de la cintura
walk	caminar
watery	acuoso
wisdom tooth	el diente de juicio
wrist	la muñeca

Some Other Useful Language Tools

Meanwhile, here are some tools that will help you navigate in the medical arena with minimal Spanish or none at all.

- Carry an English/Spanish dictionary with you. Standalone electronic gadgets are nearly useless, but a book is very helpful.
- A real translation application on a smartphone can be helpful too. But remember that no one likes to wait while you struggle with an unfamiliar device. At least if you use a book, they know you know how to use it and you aren't wasting their time.
- Many Spanish sites have an "English" option on the main menu to see a translated version.
- Google's Language Tools, can be useful, although the translations can be awkward and shouldn't be relied upon for important documents like resumes or formal correspondence.
- "Translated search" allows you to enter a search term in any language and see where that term occurs on the web in a number of other languages including English and Spanish.
- Copy and paste or type what you want to translate into the "Translate text" field and Google will give an approximate translation. Make sure you select both the source language and the one you want the result in.
- If you enter a single word into the "Translate text" field, Google will both translate the word and offer you a button that plays the translation aloud so you can hear the pronunciation.
- You can translate whole web pages by entering the URL you want to translate into the "Translate web site" field. If you travel around that website, Google will continue to translate it for you.

Coping with Alcoholism in Mexico

AA (Alcoholics Anonymous) Meetings in Mexico

It is important for many people to know that there are lots of Alcoholics Anonymous meetings in Mexico in both English and Spanish. If you or family members are dealing with alcoholism, you will be welcome at any meeting, even if the meetings are in Spanish and you speak only English. The format is so similar you will recognize what is going on and the support transcends language.

Clearly, just as in many parts of the world, alcoholism in Mexico is a relatively common, yet highly destructive health issue. Many tourists and expats arrive in Mexico knowing about their alcoholism and for them, attending AA meetings is something they know is essential to their wellbeing.

For others, particularly for expat retirees, the problem of increased drinking and alcoholism may be revealed or exacerbated by the social isolation they may encounter in Mexico, especially if they don't speak Spanish. So, learning Spanish and having expat friends (especially during the holiday's) can be critically important. But if you are using your circle of expat friends as a source of drinking buddies to binge with, you are in trouble and need to not only learn Spanish, but to stop drinking. [*See Expat Groups for Medical Referrals & Social Networking*]

However, no matter how, why or when drinking becomes a problem for you or your family member, sobriety with the support of other AA members is the solution.

While there are Mexican Alcoholics Anonymous meetings in Spanish in every town of any size in Mexico, English-language AA meetings can also be found in many towns and cities now, and not just the ones with large expat communities. Here are some of the ones with regular meetings in English:

Acapulco
Alamos
Baja (numerous)
Cabo San Lucas
Cancun
Cozumel
Cuernavaca
Guadalajara
Guanajuato
Ixtapa and Zihuatenejo
Lake Chapala
Loreto
Maxatlan
Merida
Mexico City Oaxaca

144

Playa del Carmen
Puerto Escondido
Puerto Penasco (Rocky Point)
Puerto Vallarta
San Carlos
San Jose de Cabo
San Miguel de Allende
Sonora

Although meeting times and locations in Mexico are subject to change, you will find a good starting place would be either Alcoholics Anonymous International's downloadable list or—for more reliable information about meetings in English—on Mexico Mike's website. (Mexico Mike provided the experience, wisdom and much of the information this section. He encourages its wide copyright-free distribution.)

AA is very visible in Mexico. Look for the AA symbol of a triangle inside a circle, usually on a blue background, often on a sign attached to a building. Meetings are usually at 8:00 or 8:30 PM. Even if you don't speak Spanish, you will be welcome and often asked to speak. This is true all over the world: the language of AA is truly universal—so don't hesitate to go and speak in either language. You'll be glad you did.

Meetings last an hour and a half and there are often refreshments and birthdays are celebrated like they are in the US. There are both hard-core groups in institutional settings known as "Grupo de 24 Horas" and those that are more casual. You should be prepared for longer meetings with long, emotional orations and lots of slang.

Most AA meetings in Mexico welcome those who are recovering from drug addiction and most also welcome the family members of alcoholics. Some even have AAnon groups to support family. There are many more cities and pueblas with AA meetings that are not in English. You can find a meeting near you online.[95] There are Narcotics Anonymous (NA) meetings in some parts of Mexico as well.[96]

Watching for Hidden Alcohol in Mexico

Mexico Mike suggests these additional tips to help you negotiate the social landscape in Mexico and avoiding alcohol:

- Forget the myth that it is a shooting offense to refuse a drink offered by a Mexican. You can refuse anything you want if you do it politely. Mexicans are only offering to share something with you because they are being polite. If you simply say *"No gracias, no bebo cerveza* (tequila, ron or simply alcohol) *pero quisiero un refresco,"* you'll probably get a soft drink and no one will be offended.
- If a guy insist that you have a drink with him, be as polite as possible and just as insistent. Plead illness, medication or whatever you are comfortable with. Saying *"Soy alérgico a alcohol,"* sometimes does the trick, but saying you are an alcoholic usually elicits a blank stare. If all else fails, get up and walk away. Offending a drunk does not rank as a punishable offense in any country and you have to remember what's really important.
- Be especially careful ordering tonic water or *agua quina* in bars or restaurants. You'll often end up with gin and tonic because the waiter thought you didn't speak Spanish well enough.
- When asking if a dish has alcohol in it, be sure to ask if it has wine, too. Wine is often not considered alcohol by waiters. They will say, "Oh no, there is no alcohol, only a little wine." I subscribe to the school that alcohol does not cook out. Even if you don't believe that to be true at home, believe it in Mexico. Trust me.
- Coffees with fancy names like "Sexy, Spanish or German" are suspect. If the price is more than plain coffees, then it is a booze drink.
- It is rare, but I've had Amaretto poured over flan, the great dessert. Always use the sniff test before eating anything with a sauce on it. If you accidentally imbibe something with booze, spit it out and don't worry about it. It happens to the best. Just don't take a second swig or taste and forget about it.
- If you have an AA medallion or ring, wear it. You'll be surprised at the people you'll meet.

Complaints About Medical Care

It is Important to Report Malpractice

Although it is unlikely, if you have a bad experience with medical care in Mexico, you should register complaints with both the consumer protection agency, the *Procuraduría Federal de Consumidor* (Profeco) and the medical organization that arbitrates medical concerns and conflicts, the *Comisión Nacional de Arbitraje Medico* (Conamed). It is important to register any complaint so that the Mexican authorities have the opportunity to correct the situation and other consumer/patients are protected.

Procuraduría Federal de Consumidor (PROFECO)

The Profeco address is:

Procuraduría Federal del Consumidor [97]
Av. José Vasconcelos No. 208,
6° Piso, Col. Condesa
C.P. 06140, México D. F.

You must submit the following information:

- A brief letter (1-page maximum, preferably, typed) stating the following:
- Supplier's name, address, phone, e-mail or other contact information, description of the facts that explain the reason for your complaint, date of purchase, cost of the product or service, amount you are claiming, your name and signature.
- Copy of your ID (Passport or Driver's License)
- Copy of your contract or payment invoice
- Copy of your bills, credit card slips or receipts as evidence of your payments
- Copy of all the documents available to support the complaint.

The Comisión Nacional de Arbitraje Medio (CONAMED)

CONAMED describes their organization as, "a public institution that offers alternative means for the solution of controversies between users and suppliers of health services, and promotes quality health services to guarantee patients safety, using procedures that operate under national and international quality standards." Initial contact with Comisión Nacional de Arbitraje Medico can be made via electronic mail that originates on their website. [98]

The Dark Side of Mexican Medical Care

Here are the things we've discovered that may be of concern in Mexico. These are not common situations, but you need to be aware of potential problems and what to do about them.

Uncertain Emergency Response

Our local IMSS hospital recently announced they had new ambulances. However, when faced with a recent emergency, we discovered that those new ambulances were reserved to transport patients between various IMSS facilities. Who would have thought? We ended up calling the Red Cross.

Our previous residence in the countryside was not served by a local ambulance service at all. Ambulances had to be summoned from the nearest city, over a half-hour away. Compound that with the crazy addresses in much of Mexico. Many people draw maps with the directions to their houses, but that system is useless in an emergency. You need to have clear verbal directions in Spanish and make sure the driver takes your phone number in case he or she get lost along the way.

Ambulances in Mexico are not always the mobile emergency rooms they are in the USA. There may be no equipment to speak of onboard, no highly trained paramedic at your side. Our Red Cross ambulance didn't have a chair designed to take patients down stairs. A dining room chair had to stand in. They did get us to the hospital safely.

There are private ambulance services but they expect to be paid in cash at the time of service so you really need to always have adequate cash on hand. You should also know precisely the hospital you want to be taken to. [*See Payouts from Hospitals*]

It is a good idea to actually visit your local ambulance service, take a look at their vehicles and equipment and discover what they charge in an emergency.

Medical Quackery

Although not a common problem, beware of physicians who are not displaying their *cedula* (license). [*See Licensing of Medical Professionals*] If a doctor claims an area of specialty, they should also display their board certification by the appropriate medical board. If you suspect that you might be seeing a forgery, or you would like to verify board membership, contact the medical board directly. [*See Medical Board Certification & Medical Specialties*] Report instances of quackery or malpractice to the authorities. [*See Complaints About Medical Care*]

We include in this warning unqualified expats or other native English speakers who are either posing as trained physicians or who may actually be physicians who have lost their license in the USA or Canada, or perhaps have simply failed to register with Mexico's INM. You can discover if a doctor has a license by entering their name online on the government's website.[99]

Payouts from Hospitals

Mexico has widespread, loose systems of petty graft and payouts of many types including kickbacks by hospitals to hotels, ambulance services and doctors for patient referrals. This isn't viewed as a big deal in Mexico—rather more like people performing services commonly expect to be tipped. However, if you are taken in an ambulance to a facility that has less-than-stellar capabilities while driving past the better option, this may obviously have serious impact for you.

There are hospitals that disavow this practice, sometimes to their own detriment. However, if you are clear about whom your physician is and where you wish to be taken you will reduce this likelihood. This assumes you have done your homework and know your doctor's hospital affiliation or his or her hospital recommendation and/or the circumstances aren't so life-threatening that you need the most rapid intervention available.

Churning for Increased Billing

This problem is not unique to Mexico. There are a few unethical medical practitioners who are more interested in "repeat business" than in curing the patient. The joke about paying for your doctor's children's college tuition can literally be true. If you are being asked to visit the doctor repeatedly for treatment, particularly if you sense that these visits are not essential to your health—or improving it in some critical way—we recommend that you pursue a second opinion.

Not Being Released from the Hospital

Similar to churning for increased billing, there are rare times when hospital administrators, especially in small private hospitals, may keep a patient longer than necessary, fail to provide a final billing and otherwise delay a patient's departure. It is highly recommended that you do NOT give a hospital your credit or debit card upon admission. Tell the hospital that you will pay in cash when you are given a final bill upon your release. If you must give a hospital your credit information, call your bank or credit card company, explain the situation so your account isn't drained, approve incremental payments only when you have been given a bill. Check the bill item by item and contest questionable charges.

If you feel you are being held unreasonably or taken advantage of, contact your medical evacuation insurance provider if you have this type of insurance and tell them what is going on. They have experience handling these situations and will tell you exactly what to do. If you don't have evacuation insurance, call your country's embassy or the nearest consulate, tell them what is going on and ask for their help. [*See Embassies & Consulates in Mexico*]

Overly Expensive, Outdated or Unnecessary Surgery

If you are being encouraged to pursue a major surgery or an expensive course of treatment—particularly when you have heard only one physician's opinion—then your best insurance against medical or financial malpractice is to get a second opinion. Sometimes information about less expensive, less invasive, more current or safer options is withheld to encourage you to take a more expensive or profitable route.

While this kind of abuse is rare, there is no reason not to guard your health and your pocketbook by confirming the wisdom of any physician you are working with by getting a second opinion. Legitimate doctors understand the value of consulting with other professionals and will not be threatened by your pursuit of your own best health options. Getting a second opinion is always a good idea.

Popular Travel Destinations with Marginal Care

The Mexican medical system is primarily intended to serve Mexicans where they live, not foreign tourists where they vacation. Some popular tourist destinations may have inadequate, antiquated or highly expensive medical systems. There are notable exceptions to this of course, but if you become ill or injured in a resort area, you may find that you need to seek treatment in a more populated city, hopefully nearby, once you are in a stable condition.

Another factor may be how far south you are traveling. While border areas frequently have facilities that cater to the medical needs of foreigners and medical tourists, and Mexico City and other large cities have excellent care, isolated pueblos in poor southern states may be unable to provide adequate care for complex, life-threatening conditions.

There is a relatively new chain of hospitals, Amerimed Hospitals, that has identified the need for better care at tourist destinations and is addressing it by building facilities that offer round-the-clock care in resort areas with English-speaking staff. So far, they have hospitals in Baja California Sur, Los Cabos, Puerto Vallarta, Cancun, Cabo San Lucas and Los Barriles. However, as tourists are always seeking new isolated destinations and remote beaches, there isn't always going to be a hospital at hand where they want to visit.

If you have a serious medical condition such as heart problems or diabetes, you may want to choose your vacation destination in part based on the availability of care and get a medical checkup and hear your doctor's advice before taking off for remote locations.

Your Regular Medical Insurance Won't Be Taken

It is highly unlikely that your homegrown health insurance will be taken, even in an emergency. You many not have any coverage in Mexico at all or may be reimbursed by your carrier (only for emergency care in some instances) hospitals and doctors will not bill your insurance for you, although you often can bill them yourself. You will be asked for a credit card or cash when services are delivered and if you cannot get credit, you will be expected to call relatives until you ransom yourself. You should consider other insurance options while traveling or if you relocate to Mexico. [*See Paying for Health Care in Mexico*]

Safety is Not First in Mexico

While Mexico has made tremendous progress in health practices, safety concerns lag behind. Building of infrastructure such as sidewalks (frequently non-existent), cobble streets, broken curbs, uneven pavement and non-standard stair heights contribute to twisted ankles and broken bones.

You must exercise caution with every step in Mexico no matter where you are. And since Americans and Canadians have bodies that are trained over the years to expect to walk on nearly flawless surfaces and to find footfalls on stairways to be evenly spaced, it takes a certain amount of consciously re-training your body to become more alert. Expect to move more slowly and carefully in Mexico.

Car safety is another serious issue. The rules of the road are only loosely followed and roadways and signage may not exist at all or can be difficult for non-locals to understand. Traffic in Mexico City alternates between gridlock levels of congestion and breakneck high-performance driving and should be avoided until you've actually seen what you'd be getting involved in and decided if it is worth risking your life or not when busses and taxis are more likely to get you to your destination intact.

There are Mobility Issues

Since walking around Mexico takes some adjustment for able-bodied people, it is undoubted harder for the elderly and people with disabilities, particularly those using wheelchairs or walkers. People tend to be very kind and generous. For example, it isn't unusual to see young men come to the aid of wheelchair users who needs help managing a stairway or curb. But by and large, many parts of Mexico are not wheelchair friendly.

Of course, there are people who manage rich lives with disabilities in all parts of Mexico. In cities mobility is better if you can drive since valet parking and handicapped parking places are available many places. Taxis are common and cheap when compared to the US or Canada and drivers will typically help get a wheelchair in and out of the cab. But over all, you will want to explore your options carefully and perhaps begin to study the experiences of others through websites in order to have the best possible experiences traveling or living in Mexico. [*See Appendix P: Accessible Travel Resources*]

Feeling Pressure to Accept Bad Alternatives

While this is not just a phenomena of medicine in Mexico, it is still of concern. People who have been given a diagnosis for a terminal illness or who have been told they require a medical intervention that is beyond their reach financially, are vulnerable to pursuing high-risk and/or high-priced treatments proposed as alternatives.

While it is everyone's right to seek healthcare alternatives that offer relief—and there are a number of promising alternatives available in Mexico that are not yet approved in the USA or

Canada—you should be aware that there is a lot of variation in the efficacy and safety of many "new" or experimental treatments. [*See Experimental & Non-Approved Treatments*]

You have to be realistic by asking hard questions of yourself and medical practitioners and carefully evaluate the risks and potential downside as well as the potential improvement that might be had. It is one thing for a treatment to be ineffective. It is another for a treatment to leave you in worse condition than when you started. If this is a possibility, you need to know.

Please consider that your quality of life is important, especially when you know that time with friends and family may be limited and ultimately spending time with them may be more important to you than seeking a radical treatment far from home that may only extend your life a few weeks longer. Some treatments could negatively impact the comfort you can take being with those you love during the end of your life.

Remember also that hope, desperation or wishful thinking can cloud your ability to make good judgments. In those circumstances where a treatment seems promising to you, it may be helpful to have friends, family members or trusted professionals help you research the alternatives and to use them as a sounding board in order to arrive at the best decision regarding experimental treatment for your unique situation.

Appendicitis Mistaken for "Tourista"

Travelers the world over are sometime beset with traveler's stomach: intestinal infections or food poisoning. This can be the result of food that is improperly cleaned, prepared or stored, or that is simply too old. Or it may be some local version of a stomach flu. Sometimes the fault is not with how the food is handled so much as exposure to locally common microscopic organisms for which the traveler has no natural immunity. However, the symptoms of "*tourista*," as this condition is typically called in Mexico, are also very similar to adult appendicitis and can be easily mistaken.

Fewer than half of all adults over age 50 will have the symptoms most strongly associated with appendicitis: sever right-sided abdominal pain (especially with movement), aversion to food and fever.

If you are experiencing diarrhea, mild to moderate diffused abdominal pain, low-grade fever and fatigue for more than three days, by all means seek a medical examination. Be sure to tell your doctor that you have not had your appendix removed.

Rather than immediately removing the appendix, it is common for doctors in Mexico, as in many other parts of the world these days, to treat appendicitis with a course of antibiotics followed up with careful observation. However, an infected appendix may require surgery and the older we are, the more serious such a surgery could be. Early intervention may help. So, do not assume that every intestinal condition is "*tourista*." See a doctor and have it checked.

About the Author

Monica Rix Paxson is an award-winning and best-selling author and the publisher for Relentlessly Creative Books.[100] Although she has written a number of non-fiction books, science, especially the environment and medicine, is her passion.

Her planetary science book, *Dead Mars, Dying Earth* won a Benjamin Franklin Award as a best science/environmental book and her Internet writing on the environment was commended as Best Science website by The National Science Foundation, The Andrews W. Mellon Foundation and Microsoft Corp.

Monica blogs frequently on the subject of medical care in Mexico and related topics for Mexperience.com. She is also co-author, with husband Luis Felipe Garcia Perez, of *The English Speaker's Guide to Doctors & Hospitals in Mexico*, a directory of English-speaking medical providers, and companion to this book. Her books are available in pdf format at Mexperience.com's online ebookstore and in print and Kindle versions on Amazon.com.

Monica and her husband live happily the the "perfect" climate and beautiful scenery of Cuernavaca, Morelos in the mountains of central Mexico.

Appendix A: The English Speaker's Guide to Doctors & Hospitals in Mexico

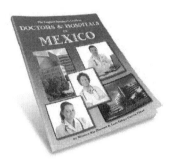

Mexico has one of the most interesting and unexpectedly enlightened medical systems in the world. From its long and ancient history of herbalism and healing, to today's modern health centers which offer patients the latest technologies in medical science, doctors and hospitals in Mexico save lives and make whole many of us who seek help because we are ill or injured.

While the supply is plentiful (Mexico counts over 4,000 private and public hospitals and countless medical doctors and dentists), there remains a unique challenge for foreigners seeking healthcare services here. When the need for medical care arises, we are filled with questions: Where do I go to find the care that I need? Where can we find a doctor or dentist that understands English? Where is the nearest specialist? Where do we go in an emergency?

To help foreign residents and frequent visitors to Mexico connect with medical services locally, a new guide has been published: *The English Speaker's Guide to Doctors & Hospitals in Mexico.*

The guide is written and edited by Monica Rix Paxson (who authored the highly popular *The English Speaker's Guide to Medical Care in Mexico*) and husband and co-author Luis Felipe Garcia Perez. This latest title offers a comprehensive and fully up-to-date directory of English-speaking medical resources: doctors, hospitals, clinics, dentists and specialists in Mexico. The guide covers medical practices and practitioners at over 90 different locations across the country, including all the major towns and cities, and many of the secondary towns and small settlements near them.

The doctors and hospitals in this guide have been recommended by sources trusted by the authors. The vast majority of physicians listed speak English (although proficiency will vary). In instances where doctors only speak Spanish this is noted alongside the entry.

This guide offers a practical information resource that can be used to find medical care services in the place or places where you are, or intend to be. The book is available in pdf format at Mexperience.com.[101] It is also available in print and Kindle versions on Amazon.com and through the publisher's website.[102]

Appendix B: Medical History Form

INTERNATIONAL TRAVEL MEDICAL HISTORY FORM

Your Name:_____ Date of birth:_____ Age:_____ Gender: M   F

Address:_____City:_____ZIP_____Phone:_____

Your Pharmacy:_____Address:_____Phone:_____

Your medical doctor:_____Address:_____Phone:_____

MEDICAL HISTORY: Please circle "yes" or "no" to the following questions **(attach additional pages if necessary)**:

1. Have you ever had severe reactions to immunizations/vaccinations?   Yes   No   If yes, please describe:_____

2. Are you being treated for leukemia, lymphoma, cancer or any other malignant disease: Yes   No

3. Do you have a history of deficiency of the immune system?   Yes   No

4. Do you had medical treatment for any blood disorder?   Yes   No

5. Do you have any existing medical condition such as diabetes, heart disease or pulmonary disease? Yes   No   If yes, please list /:describe:_____

6. Do you have a history of kidney disease?   Yes   No

7. Do you have a history of psychiatric disorder? Yes   No   OR Severe Depression? Yes   No

8. Do you have a history of seizures?   Yes   No

9. Are you pregnant; suspect you may be pregnant or trying to become pregnant? Yes   No

10. Are you breastfeeding? Yes   No

11. Do you have any allergies to the following? (Circle all that apply)

    Eggs   Neomycin   Antibiotics   Mercury (thinerosal)   Bee Stings   Streptomycin   Polymyxin B

If yes, please describe the reaction:_____

12. Are there any other drugs to which you have had an allergic reaction?   Yes   No   If yes, please list and describe:_____

13. List all of the medications you are currently taking. Include medications for allergies and skin problems.   _____

14. **TRAVEL INFORMATION**: Departure date:_____   Return date:_____

15. Please indicate the countries you will be visiting (attach additional pages if necessary):

Destination	Where will you stay	Length of stay:	Rural Travel or camping
			Yes No
			Yes No
			Yes No
			Yes No

16. Please mark all the vaccines you have had including the date of vaccination:

	Date			Date			Date
❑ Typhoid injection		❑ Yellow Fever		❑ Japanese Encephalitis	
❑ Typhoid oral		❑ Meningococcal		❑ Measles/Mumps/Rubella	
❑ Hepatitis A		❑ Immune Globulin		❑ Tetanus Diphtheria	
❑ Hepatitis B		❑ Polio		❑ Rabies	
❑ Malaria drug (name of drug)				❑ Varicella (Chicken Pox	

*Client Signature:*_____   *Reviewed by:*_____*Date:*_____

Appendix C: Medical Specialties & Medical Boards

Allergy (Also see Immunology)

Colegio Mexicano de Pediatras Especialistas en Inmunología Clínica y Alergia [103]

Colegio Mexicano de Inmunología Clínica y Alergia, A. C. [104]

Anesthesiology

Consejo Mexicana de Anestesiología [105]

Angioloy & Vascular Surgery

Consejo Mexican de Angiología y Cirugía Vascular, A. C. [106]

Audiologists

La Asociacion Mexicana de Comunicación, Audiología, Otoneurología A.C. [107]

Cardiology

Sociedad Mexicana de Cardiologia [108]

Asociación Nacional de Cardiólogos de México [109]

Colorectal (Also see Surgery, Colorectal)

Colegio Mexicano de Especialistas en Coloproctologia, A.C. [110]

Colposcopy & Cervical (Also see Gynecology & Obstetrics)

Asociación Mexicana de Colposcopía y Patología Cervical, A.C. [111]

Critical Care

Consejo Mexicano de Medicina Crítica, A.C. [112]

Dermatology

Fundacion Mexicana para la Dermatologia, A.C. [113]

Consejo Mexicano de Dermatología [114]

Academia Mexicana de Dermatología, A.C. [115]

Emergency Medicine

Consejo Mexicano de Medicina de Urgencias, A.C. [116]

Endrocrinologists

Consejo Mexicano de Endocrinología, A.C. [117]

Family Medicine

Consejo Mexicano de Certificación en Medicina Familiar A.C. [118]

Colegio Mexicano de Medicina Familiar, A.C. [119]

Gastroenterology

Consejo Mexicano de Gastroenterología [120]

Asociación Mexicana de Gastroenterología [121]

Genetics

Consejo Mexicano de Genética [122]

Geriatrics

Consejo Mexicano de Geriatría, A.C. [123]

Gynecology & Obstetrics (Also see Colposcopy & Cervical)

Federacion Mexicana de Colegios de Obstetricia y Ginecologia, A.C. [124]

Consejo Mexicano de Ginecología y Obstetricia, A.C. [125]

Hematology

Consejo Mexicano de Hematología, A.C. [126]

Infectious Diseases

Consejo Mexicano de Certificación en Infectología, A.C. [127]

Immunology (Also see Allergies, Pediatrics)

La Sociedad Mexicana de Inmunología [128]

Colegio Mexicano de Pediatras Especialistas en Inmunología Clínica y Alergia [129]

Internal Medicine

Consejo Mexicano de Medicina Interna, A.C. [130]

Nephrology

Consejo Mexicano de Nefrología, A.C. [131]

Neurology

Academia Mexicana de Neurología A. C. [132]

Consejo Mexicano de Neurologia [133]

Neurophysiology

Consejo Mexicano de Neurofisiología Clínica, A.C. [134]

Neurosurgery (See Surgery, Neurosurgery)

Nuclear Medicine

Consejo Mexicano de Médicos Nucleares [135]

Obstetrics (See Gynecology & Obstetrics)

Occupational Medicine

Consejo Nacional Mexicano de Medicina del Trabajo, A.C. [136]

Oncology

Sociedad Mexicana de Oncología [137]

Consejo Mexicano de Oncología, A.C. [138]

Ophthalmology

Sociedad Mexicana de Oftalmología [139]

Consejo Mexicano De Oftalmología [140]

Oral & Maxillofacial Surgery (See Surgery, Maxillofacial)

Orthopedic (See Surgery, Orthopedic)

Otolaryngology

Consejo Mexicano de Otorrinolaringología y Cirugía de Cabeza y Cuello [141]

Pathology

Consejo Mexicano de Patología Clinica y Medicina de Laboratorio [142]

Consejo Mexicano de Médicos Anatomopatólogos, A.C. [143]

Pediatrics

Consejo Mexicano de Certificación en Pediatría A.C. [144]

Colegio Mexicano de Pediatras Especialistas en Inmunología Clínica y Alergia [145]

Physical Therapy & Rehabilitation

Consejo Mexicano de Medicina de Rehabilitación [146]

Plastic Surgery (See Surgery, Plastic)

Pulmonology (Pneumology)

Consejo Nacional de Neumología, A.C. [147]

Proctology (See Surgery, Colorectal)

Psychiatry

Consejo Mexicano de Psiquiatría, A.C. [148]

Psychology

Sociedad Mexicana de Psicologia [149]

Public Health

Sociedad Mexicana de Salud Publica [150]

Radiology & Imaging (Also see Nuclear Medicine)

La Federación Mexicana de Radiología e Imagen (FMRI) [151]

Consejo Mexicano de Radiología e Imagen, A.C. [152]

Rehabilitation (See Physical Medicine & Rehabilitation)

Respiratory Medicine (See Pulmonology)

Rheumatology

Consejo Mexicano de Reumatología, A.C. [153]

Sports Medicine

Consejo Nacional de Medicina del Deporte, A.C. [154]

Surgery, Colorectal

Sociedad Mexicana de Cirujanos de Recto y Colon [155]

Consejo Mexicano de especialistas en Coloproctología, A.C. [156]

Surgery, Chest

Consejo Nacional de Cirugía del Tórax, A.C. [157]

Surgery, General

Asociación Mexicana de Cirugía General [158]

Consejo Mexicano de Cirugía General, A.C. [159]

Surgery, Head & Neck (See Otolaryngology)

Surgery, Maxillofacial

Consejo Mexicano de Cirugía Oral y Maxilofacial, A.C. [160]

Surgery, Neurosurgery (Also see Neurology)

Sociedad Mexicana de Cirugía Neurológica, A.C. [161]

Surgery, Orthopedic

Colegio Mexicano de Ortopedia y Traumatología A.C. [162]

Federación Mexicana de Colegios de Ortopedia y Traumatología, A.C. [163]

Surgery, Pediatric

Sociedad Mexicana de Cirugía Pediátrica [164]

Consejo Mexican de Cirugía Pediátrica [165]

Surgery, Plastic

Asociación Mexicana de Cirugía Plástica, Estética y Reconstructiva [166]

Consejo Mexicano de Cirugía Plástica Estética y Reconstructiva, A.C. [167]

Surgery, Vascular (See Angiology)

Tramatology (See Surgery, Orthopedic)

Urology

Consejo Nacional Mexicano de Urología, A.C. [168]

Appendix D: USA, Canadian & UK Consulates in Mexico

City/Consulate	Telephone	Hours

Acapulco

US	744-469-0556 744-484-0300	M-F, 10am–2pm
Canada	744-484-1305	M-F, 9am–5pm
Assistance for Other Consulates	744-484-1735 744-481-2533	M-F, 9am–3pm

Cabo San Lucas

US	624-143-3566	M-F, 9am–2pm

Cancún

US	988-883-0272	M-F, 9am–2pm
Canada	988-883-3360	M-F, 9am–5pm
United Kingdom	988-881-0100	M-F, 9am–2pm

Cozumel

US	987 -872-4574	M-F, 12pm–2pm

Guadalajara

US	33-3825-2700 33-3826-6549 33-3826-5553	M-F, 8am–4:30pm (emergencies)
Canada	33-3615-6215 33-3615-6266 33-3615-6270	M-F, 8:30am–2pm
United Kingdom	33-642-9875	M-F, 8:30am–3pm

Hermosillo

US	622-217-1205	M-F, 8am–4:30pm
	622-217-2375	
	622-217-2555	

Ixtapa/Zihuatanejo

US	044-755-557-1106	M-F, 1pm–5pm
	(emergency mobile)	

Mazatlán

US	669-916-5889	M-F, 9am–1pm
Canada	669-913-7320	M-F, 9am–1pm

Mérida

US	999-925-5011	M-F, 7:30am-4pm

Mexico City

US	55-5080-2000	M-F, 8:30am–1:30pm
		3pm–6pm
Canada	55-5724-7900	M-F, 8:45am–5:15pm
United Kingdom	55-242-8500	M-F, 2:30pm–9:30pm
		(Winter)
		M-F, 3:30pm–8:30pm
		(Summer)

Monterrey

US	81-8345-2120	M-F, 8am–12pm
Canada	81-8344-3200	M-F, 9am–1:30pm,
		2:30pm–5:30pm
United Kingdom	81-8356-5359	M-F, 10am-4pm

Oaxaca City

US	951-514-3054 951-516-2853	M-F, 9am–3pm
Canada	951-513-3777	M-F, 11am–2pm

Puerto Vallarta

US	322-222-0069	M-F, 10am–2pm
Canada	322-293-0098 322-293-0099	M-F, 9am–3pm

San José de Cabo

Canada	624-142-4333	M-F, 9am -1pm

San Miguel de Allende

US	415-152-2357 415-152-1588	M-F, 9am–1pm
Canada	(no phone)	M-F, 9am–1pm

Tijuana

US	664-622-7400, 664-692-2154	M-F, 8am–4:30pm
Canada	664-684-0461	M-F, 9am–1pm
United Kingdom	664-686-5320, 664-681-7323	M-F, 9am–2pm

Appendix E: JCI Accredited Hospitals in Mexico

The American British Cowdray (ABC) Medical Center IAP - Observatorio Campus

Mexico City, Mexico
Program: Hospital
First Accredited: December 2008

The American British Cowdray (ABC) Medical Center IAP - Sante Fe Campus

Mexico City, Mexico
Program: Hospital
First Accredited: December 2008

Assisteo Mexico S.A. de C.V.

Mexico City, Mexico
Program: Home Medical Assistants
First Accredited: March 2012
(not on current list)

Centro Oncologico de Chihuahua

Chihuahua, Mexico
Program: Ambulatory Care
First Accredited, April 2014

Christus Muguerza Alta Especialidad

Monterrey, Mexico
Program: Hospital
First Accredited: July 2007
(not on current list)

Clinica Cumbres Chihuahua

Chihuahua, Mexico
Program: Ambulatory Care
First Accredited: 23 April 2008

Hospital Angeles Valle Oriente

Nuevo Leon, Mexico
Program: Hospital
(not on current list)

Hospital CIMA Chihuahua

Chihuahua, Mexico
Program: Ambulatory Care
First Accredited: August 2012
(not on current list)

Hospital CIMA Hermosillo

Hermosillo, Sonora, Mexico
Program: Hospital
First Accredited: December 2008
(not on current list)

Hospital CIMA Monterrey

San Pedro Garza Garcia, N.L., Mexico
Program: Hospital
First Accredited: December 2008
(not on current list)

Hospital Galenia

Cancun, Mexico
Program: Hospital
First Accredited: October 2012
http://hospitalgalenia.com/

Hospital Mexico Americano, SC

Guadalajara, Jalisco, Mexico
Program: Hospital
First Accredited: March 2010
(not on current list)

Hospital San Jose Tec de Monterrey

Monterrey, Nuevo Leon, Mexico
Program: Hospital
First Accredited: December 2007
(not on current list)

Hospital Y Clinica OCA, S.A. de C.V.

Monterrey, Nuevo Leon, Mexico
Program: Hospital
First Accredited: September 2008
(not on current list)

Obesity Control Center (Cyntar SC)

Program: Ambulatory Care
Tijuana, Mexico
First Accredited: January 2016

Médica Sur S.A.B de C.V.

Mexico City, Mexico
Program: Hospital
First Accredited: May 2014

Appendix F: Private Hospitals by State & City

Acapulco de Juárez

Acapulco de Juárez

OHA Sucursal Hospital Angeles Querétaro

Bernardino Del Razo #21, Ensueño
01 442 216 97 17

Aguascalientes

Aguascalientes

Central Medico Quirurgica de Aguascalientes S.A. de C. V.

Rep. del Peru No. 112, Las Americas
01(49)10-6120/7820-4 / 01(49)10-61-27/78-2

Baja California

Mexicali

Hospital Almater S.A. de C.V. Madero No. 1060, Nueva

01(686)552-52-84/5 / 01(686)553-31-50/5
patriciameza@almater.com
www.almater.com

Hospital Mexico-Americano de B.C. S.A. C.V.

Reforma y Calle B 1000, Segunda Seccion
01 686 552 23 00 / 01 686 552-29-42
mercadotecnia@hospitalhispanoamericano.com
www.hospitalhispanoamericano.com

Hospital de la Mujer, S.A. de C.V.

Circuito Brasil No. 82, Parque Industrial El Alamo

Centro Medico Hospital del Prado, S.A. de C.V.

Bugambilias No. 50, Del Prado
01 664 681-49-00 al 0 / 01 664 681-65-40
trasplanterenal@hotmail.com

Hospital Centro Medico Nova S.A. de C.V.

Guadalupe Victoria No. 9308 1 y 4, Zona Rio
01(664)634-61-50 co / 01(664)634-36-37
hnova@telnor.net

Centro Medico Excel S.C.

Av. Paseo de los Heroes No. 2507, Zona del Rio
01 664 634 34 34 / 01 664 634 22 90
centroexcel@hotmail.com

Hospital Oasis

Paseo Playas No. 19 Secc. Monumental, Playas de Tijuana
01 664 631 61 61 / 01 664 631 61 62
hospital@oasisofhope.com

Instituto Nefrologico de Tijuana S.A. de C.V.

Mision San Ignacio No. 10616, Zona Rio, 63 47 408

OHA Sucursal Hospital Angeles Tijuana

Av. Paseo de los Heroes No. 10999, Zona Rio
01 664 635 19 00 ext / 01 664 635 19 15

Chihuahua

Chihuahua

Servicios Hospitalarios de Mexico S.A. de C.V.

Haciendas del Valle No. 7120, Plaza Las Haciendas
01 614 439 27 00 / 01 614 429 37 23
jvaldes@hospitalcima.com.mx
www.hospitalcima.com.mx

Juárez

Clinica del Parque S.A. de C.V.

Pedro Leal Rodriquez No. 1802, Centro
01 614 439 79 79 / 01 614 439 79 20
clinicaparque@infosel.net.mx
www.hcp.com.mx

Poliplaza Medica (Hospitales de Juarez)

Pedro Rosales de León No. 7510,
Fuentes del Valle
617 32 00 / 617 32 00
alfredosd@gmail.com
http://www.poliplaza.com/

Hospitales del Valle S.A. de C.V.

Avenida HerHands Escobar #3213, La Playa
611 22 22
alfredosd@gmail.com

OHA Sucursal Hospital Angeles Chihuahua

Ave. Campos Eliseos No. 9371,
Campos Eliseos

Coahuila

Saltillo

Clinica Quirurgica de la Concepcion

Blvd. Venustiano Carranza No. 4036, Villa Olimpica
0184-4427-3040 cel. / 0 01(84) 16-25-62

Hospital Muguerza Saltillo (Christus)

Carr. Saltillo-Monterrey Km. 4.5, Sobre Carretera
01 844 411-70-00 al / 01 844 411-70-60
bdavila@christusmuguerza.com
www.christusmuguerza.com.mx

**Clinica Hospital del Magisterio
"Prof. Niceforo Rodriguez Maldonado"**

Blvd. Antonio Cardenas #2450, Lourdes
417 31 31

Torreón

Hospital General Universitario "Dr. Joaquin del Valle Sanchez"

Av. Juarez No. 951 Ote., Centro
01(184) 713-1094

Distrito Federal (Mexico City)

Alvaro Obregón

Hospital Ingles ABC (Sucursal Observatorio)

Sur 136 N. 116 Esq. Observatorio, Las Americas
5230-8000 / 5616-570 / 5230-8037
jfeldman@abchospital.com
http://www.abchospital.com.mx/

Benito Juárez

OHA Sucursal Hospital Ángeles Metropolitano

Tlacotlalpan No. 59, Roma Sur
5265-1800 / 52 64 20 60
hector.baragan@saludangel

Hospital Infantile Privado S.A. de C.V.

Viaducto Rio Becerra No. 97, Napoles
53401010 / 53401000 / 55362257 / 56690404
jmmendoza.hip@starmedica.com
www.starmedica.com

Hospital Santa Fe S.A. de C.V.

San Luis Potosi No. 143, Roma
10844747 y 10844733 10844760
jperez@hospitalsantafe.com

www.hospitalsantafe.com.mx

Centro Medico de Especialidades de Ciudad Juarez S.A de C.V.

Av. de las Americas No. 201 Nte., Margaritas
01656 613-1311/613- / 01 656 686 01 10
cme1@infosel.net.mx
http://www.centromedicojuarez.com/

Novoinjertos (Banco de Tejidos)

Amores No. 1554, Col. Del Valle
10426199 / 10426688 / 55342222
informex@novinjertos.com.mx
www.novoinjertos.com.mx

Hospital Galenia

Av. Tulum Esquina Nizuc Manzana 1 Lote 1
Supermanzana 12, Santa Maria Sike
01 998 214 0392

Coyoacán

Hospital Merlos S.A. de C.V.

Camino Al Estadio Azteca No. 179, El Caracol
55687863 / 5650444 / 55281994
direccion@hospitalmerlos.com.mx
www.hospitalmerlos.com.mx

Hospital Hmg Coyoacan

Arbol del Fuego No. 80, El Rosario

OHA Sucursal Hospital Ángeles Clínica Londres

Durango No. 50, Roma Norte
5229-8400 / 5229-844 / 55-25-37-82
sa_garcia2000@yahoo.com

Nuevo Sanatoria Durango, S.A. de C.V.

Durango No. 296, Roma
51484646 / 51484603 / 51484603
urioste@sanatoriodurango.com
www.sanatoriodurango.com

Sanatorio Santa Catrina S.A. de C.V.

Blvd de las Rosas No. 46 Sur,
Jardines de Durango
01 618 818 22 62-63 / 01 618 818 33 90
alviver@hotmail.com

Inter-Hospitalaria, S.A. de C.V.

Centro Medico Dalinde
Tuxpan No. 25, Roma Sur
55-74-44-44

OHA Sucursal Hospital Angeles (Roma-Queretaro)

Queretaro No. 58, Roma
Gustavo Madero

Unidad de Tecnologia en Cultivo del Cinvestav

Av. Instituto Politecnico Nacional
No. 2508, San Pedro Zacatenco
57-47-70-00 Ext. 551 / 57-47-70-93
http://www.cinvestav.mx/

OHA Sucursal Lindavista

Rio Bamba No. 639,
Magdelna de las Salinas
5754.7000 ext. 2175

Magdalena Contreras, La

OHA Sucursal Hospital Ángeles Pedregal

Camino Santa Teresa No. 1055, Heroes de Padierna
5652-118 / 5652-8598 / 5449-550
ehuico@saludangeles.com

Miguel Hidalgo

Sociedad de la Beneficencia Español I.A.P.

Av. Ejercito Nacional No. 613, Granada
5255-9600 / 5203-85 5255-9665 / 5545954
ricardomz85@terra.com.mx
http://www.hespanol.com/

OHA Sucursal Hospital Ángeles Mocel

Gelati No. 29, San Miguel Chapultepec
5277-3111 / 5273-764 / 52782300/2725
aescalona@saludangeles.com
www.mediks.com

Medica Ideas, S.A. de C.V.

Blvd. Luis Donaldo Colosio Lote C-5 Mza. 02
S/N, Arboledas San Javier
017717166794

Tláhuac

Skin Theca S.A. de C.V.

Puente de Piedra 150-726, Toriello Guerra
56-66-87-82

Guanajuato

Celaya

Centro de Especialidades Medica de Celaya S.A. de C.V.

Obregon No. 209, Centro
01(461)217-72/218-47 / 01(461)245-86

León

Hospital Aranda de la Parra S.A de C.V. Hidalgo No. 329, Centro

01(477)719-71-00 / 01(47)16-49-03
gerencia@arandadelaparra.com
http://arandadelaparra.com.mx/

Jalisco

Guadalajara

Centro de Especialidades Medica de Celaya S.A. de C.V.

Obregon No. 209, Centro
01(461)217-72/218-47 / 01(461)245-86

OHA Sucursal Hospital Ángeles del Carmen

Tarascos No. 3435, Fraccionamiento
01 33 38 13 00 42 / 01 33 38 13 34 63
jmonroy@saludangeles.com
www.mediks.com

Hospital Mexico Americano S.C.

Colomos N. 2110, Ladron de Guevara
01 33 36 41-31-41 / 01 33 36 42-42-79
mex_amer@prodigy.net.mx

Hospital Santa Margarita S.A. de C.V.

Garibaldi No. 880, Sector Hidalgo
01(3)825-33-05/826- / 01(3)825-33-05/826-

Hospital San Javier S.A. de C.V.

Av. Pablo Casals No. 640 (Esq. Eulogio Parra), Prados Providencia
01 33 36 69 02 22 / 01 33 36 69 88 24
dirmed@sanjavier.com.mx
www.hospitalsanjavier.com

Hospital Country 2000

Av. Jorge Alvarez del Castillo No. 1542, Chapultepec Country
01 33 38 54 45 00 Al / 01 33 38 54 45 00 Ex
ever@hcountry.com.mx
www.hcountry.com.mx

Hospital Bernardette S.A. de C.V.

Hidalgo #930, Centro
382 54 365

Zapopan

Centro de Cirugia Avanzada Siglo XXI. S.A. de C.V.

Boulevard Puerta de Hierro No. 5150-1-B, Plaza Corporativa Zapopan
0133 38 48 4000 / 38 48 4000
archivoclinico@cmpdh.com
www.cmpdh.com

Hospital Real de San Jose

Av. Lazaro Cardenas No. 4149, Jardines de San Ignacio
0133 10 78 89 00 / 0133 10 78 89 00
joaquin.jimenez@hrsj.com.mx

Hospital de Especialidades Puerta de Hierro S.A. de C.V.

Av. Empresarios No. 150-1A, Puerta de Hierro
http://www.cmpdh.com/hospital

Centro

Clinica Santa Cruz S.A. de C.V.

Gregorio Mendez No. 707, Centro
01(93)12-13-28 / 01(93)12-36-71
faustolm@prodigy.net.mx

OHA Sucursal Hospital Angeles Villahermosa

Prol. Paseo Usumacinta S/N, Tabasco 2000
316 70 00 / 316 93 27

Cuautitlán Izcalli

Centro de Trasplantes Oncohematologicos San Rafael, S.A.

Autopista Mexico/Queretaro Km. 43,
Parque Industrial La Luz

Huixquilucan

OHA Sucursal Hospital Angeles Lomas

Vialidad de la Barranca S/N, Valle de las Palmas
52-46-50-00 ext. 5057 / 52-46-53-01
ccalihal@saludangeles.com

Metepec

Centro Medico de Toluca S.A de C.V.

Av. S.S. Juan Pablo II No. 341 Norte, Barrio de san Mateo
01(722)232-22-22 C / 01(722)232-22-23
jl.valdes@centromedicodeto.com
http://www.centromedicodetoluca.com.mx/

Servicios Medicos-Quirurgicos de Toluca S.A. de C.V.

Eulalia Peñaloza No. 233,
Federal Esq. Con Tollocan
01 722 217-7800/217- / 01 722 217-78-00
arar_ba@hotmail.com

Sanatorio Florencia S.A. de C.V.

Paseo Vicente Guerrero No. 205, Barrio San Bernardino
2144 785 / 2144 785
sll@prodigy.net.mx

Sanatorio Hidalgo de Toluca, S.A.

Avenida Hidalgo Oriente No. 411, Centro
2134299

Michoacan

Morelia

Sanatorio la Luz

General Bravo No. 55, Chapultepec Norte
01(443)315-29-66 Y / 01(443)315-29-68
contraloria@sanatoriolaluz.com
www.sanatoriolaluz.com

Hospital Star Medica S.A. de C.V.

Virrey de Mendoza No. 2000, Felix Ireta
01(443)3227700 / (443)01322701
info@starmedica.com.mx
www.starmedica.com.mx

Morelos

Cuernavaca

Instituto Mexicano de Trasplantes S.C.

Av. Alta Tension 580 2, Cantarranas
01(777)3 18 33 62 / 01(777)312 66 69
imt@prodigy.net.mx
www.imtsc.com.mx

Montmorelos

Hospital la Carlota S.C.

Camino Al Vapor No. 209, Zambrano
01(826)26350-63/331- / 01(826)267-28-59
oftalmo@um.edu.mx

Nuevo Leon

Monterrey

Hospital Christus Muguerza Monterrey S.A. de C.V.

Av. Hidalgo No. 2525 Pte., Obispado
0181 83-99-34 00 / 01 81 83 99 34 59
drguillermo70@yahoo.com

Hospital Universitario "Dr. Jose E. Gonzalez"

Av. Madero Y Gonzalitos S/N Mitras Centro
01(81) 8333-41-37 / 83 0181 / 8333-31-33 / 834
deosio@mexico.com

Hospital San José Tec de Monterrey

Fundacion Santos y de la Garza Evia, I.B.P.
Av. Ignacio Morone Prieto No. 3000, Poniente los Doctores
01(81) 8348-04-26 / 83 01(8) 347-54-13 / 348
Jvalero@itesm.mx
www.hsj.com.mx

Hospital y Clinica OCA, S.A. de C.V.

Pino Suarez No. 645 Norte, Centro
0181-8289-0380/0181 / 0181-8289-0380
danlevi@prodigy.net.mx
www.ocahospital.com

Hospital Universitario "Jose E. Gonzalez" Uanl (Banco de Tejidos)

Av. Francisco y Madero S/N, Mitras Centro
0181-8346-2071, 01-8 / 01-81-83462072
contacto@bancodeBone.org
www.bancodeBone.org

Hospital Santa Cecilia de Monterrey, S.A. de C.V.

Isaac Garza No. 200 Ote, Centro

Christus Muguerza Sur, S.A. de C.V.

Carretera Nacional No. 6501,
La Estanzuela

Christus Muguerza Conchita, S.A. de C.V.

15 de Mayo No. 1822 Pte.,
Maria Luisa

San Pedro Garza Garcia

Hospital Santa Engracia

Frida Kahlo No. 180, Valle Oriente
01(81)8368-77-77/8 / 01(81)8368-77-46
info@santaengracia.com

Oaxaca de Juárez

Oaxaca de Juárez

Hospital Reforma

Reforma No. 613, Centro

Puebla

Puebla

Hospital de la Sociedad Española de Beneficencia (Puebla)

19 Norte 1001, Jesus Garcia
0122 2293700 Ext. 1 / 0122 2293700 Ext. 1

Fundacion Tamariz Oropeza "Hospital Betania"

11 Oriente. No. 1826, Azcarate
01 22 2213 83 00 / 01 22 23672 82, 235 7
mhbetania@prodigy.net.mx

Hospital San Agustin, S.A. de C.V.

Boulevard Garcia Salinas No. 19, El Carmen

OHA Sucursal Hospital Angeles Puebla

Avenida Kepler No. 2143, Reserva Territorial Atlixcoyotl

Querétaro

Querétaro

Hospital del Niño Quemado (Queretaro)

Julio Ma. Cervantes No. 105, Colina del Cimatario
01(442)2 23-57-07 al / 01(442)2 23-57-08
queretaro_iainq@att.net.mx
www.iainq.org.mx

Centro Hospitalario B.S.A.L.A.H., S.A. de C.V.

Vasco Nuñez de Balboa #1003, Fracc. Hornos
01 744 486 34 37 jsaburton@yahoo.com.mx

Hospital San Jose de Queretaro S.A. de C.V.

Prolongacion Constituyentes No. 302, El Jacal

San Luis Potosí

San Luis Potosí

Hospital del Centro Medico del Potosi

Antonioguilar No. 155 Burocratas del Estado
01(444) 813-37-97 / 1 01 (444) 813 13 77
pasapaca@yahoo.com

Sociedad de Beneficencia Española A.C.

Av. Venustiano Carranza No. 1090, Tequisquiapan
01(48) 13-40-48 / 13-9

Hospital Lomas de San Luis Internacional

Avenida Palmira No. 600, Villas Del Pedregal

Sinaloa

Culiacan

Clinica Hospital Culiacan S.A. de C.V.

Mariano Escobedo No. 829 Ote., Centro
01(67)16 42 40

Hospital Angeles Culican

Blvd. Alfonso G. Calderon No. 2193,
Desarrollo Urbano Tres Rios

Mazatlan

Hospital Sharp de Mazatlan

Av. Rafael Buelna y Dr. Jesus Kumate S/N, Col. Las Cruces
01(67)86-56-76 al 84

Sonora

Cajeme

Hospital Privado San Jose de Ciudad Obregón S.A. de C.V.

Calle. Coahuila No. 263 Sur, Centro
01 644 4 15 02 33 y 4

Hermosillo

Centro Medico del Noroeste S.A. de C.V.

Horacio Soria Larrea y Luis D. Colosio No. 23 Centro
01(662) 217-5292 Ex. 21 / 01(662) 217-4521
mserna@clinicadelnoroeste

Hospital CIMA Hermosillo

Paseo Rio San Miguel No. 35, Proyecto Rio Sonora
01(6)259-09-00/59-0 / 01(6)259-09-99/59-0
jmojarra@rtn.uson.mx

Tamaulipas

Matamoros

Hospital General de Matamoros

Dr. Alfredo Pumarejo Lafaurie
Canales No. 800, Unidad Hogar

Reynosa

Hospital General Reynosa

"Dr. Jose Ma. Cantu Garza"
Av. Alvaro Obregon S/N, La Presa

Tampico

Hospital de Beneficencia Española (Tampico)

Av. Hidalgo No. 3909, Guadalupe
01(833) 213-54-09/21 / 01(833)213-17-84
cgarcia@bene.com
www.bene.com.mx

Veracruz

Boca del Rio

Millenium Medical Center Veracruz, S.A. de C.V.

Av. Juan Pablo II No. 148, Fracc. Costa de Oro
(22)234200

Yucatán

Mérida

Centro Medico de las Americas S.A. de C.V.

Calle 54 No. 365 Por Av. Perez Ponce, Centro
01-926-91-11

Zacatecas

Zacatecas

Hospital Santa Teresita

Calz. Garcia Salinas No. 601, Las Colinas II

Appendix G: Medical Schools in Mexico

Benemérita Universidad Autónoma de Puebla, Facultad de Medicina [169]
  Calle 13 Sur Num. 2702 y Privada de la 29 Poniente, Puebla, Pue. 72000
  Tel: +52 22 43 1447, Fax: +52 22 43 1444

Centro de Estudios Universitarios Xochicalco, Escuela de Medicina [170]
  San Francisco Num 1139, Fracc. Mision, Ensenada, B.C.N. 22830
  Tel: +52 617 785 613, Fax: +52 617 785 613

Instituto Politécnico Nacional (CICS), Centro Interdisciplinario de Ciencias de la Salud [171]
  Km. 39.5, Carretera Xochimilco Oaxtepec, Delegacion Milpa Alta, México, D.F. 12000
  Tel: +52 5 729 6300, Fax: +52 5 729 6000

Instituto Politécnico Nacional, Escuela Nacional de Medicina y Homeopatia [172]
  Guillermo Massieu Helguera Num. 239, Fraccionamiento La Escalera
  Ticoman, México, D.F. 07320
  Tel: +52 5 586 9449, Fax: +52 5 586 5524

Instituto Politécnico Nacional (ESM), Escuela Superior de Medicina [173]
  Plan de San Luis y Diaz Moron, Delegacion Miguel Hidalgo, México, D.F. 11340
  Tel: +52 5 341 3195, Fax: +52 5 729 6300

Instituto Tecnologico y de Estudios Superiores de Monterrey (ITESM), Escuela de Medicina [174]
  Avenida Ignacio Morones Prieto 3000 Poniente, Monterrey, Nuevo Leon 64710
  Tel: +52 8 348 0426, Fax: +52 8 347 5413

Universidad Anáhuac, Escuela de Medicina [175]
  Avenida Lomas Anáhuac S/N, Huixquilucan, Edo. de Méx. 52760
  Tel: +52 5 627 0210, Fax: +52 5 596 1938

Universidad Autónoma "Benito Juarez" de Oaxaca, Facultad de Medicina [176]
  Ex-Hacienda de Aquilera S/N, Oaxaca de Juárez, Oaxaca 68020
  Tel: +52 951 530 58, Fax: +52 951 530 58

Universidad Autónoma de Aguascalientes, Centro de Ciencias Biomedicas [177]
  Edificio 25, Modulo 25, Av. Universidad Km. 2
  Aguascalientes, Ags. 20100
  Tel: +52 491 107 400, Fax: +52 491 108 431

Universidad Autónoma de Baja California, Unidad Mexicali, Escuela de Medicina [178]
  Av. Misioneros s/n., Centro, Cívico Comercial, Mexicali, B.C.N. 21000

Tel: +52 65 571 622, Fax: +52 65 572 658

Universidad Autónoma de Baja California, Unidad Tijuana, Escuela de Medicina [179]

U. Universidad Ex-Ejido de Tampico, Fracc. Otay Universidad,
Tijuana, B.C.N. Tijuana, B.C.N. 22390
Tel: +52 66 821 033, Fax: +52 66 821 233

Universidad Autónoma de Campeche, Facultad de Medicina [180]

Avenida Patricio Trueva y Regil S/N, Campeche, Camp. 24090
Tel: +52 981 315 34, Fax: +52 981 315 34

Universidad Autónoma de Chiapas, Facultad de Medicina [181]

10a. Avenida Sur y Calle Central, Tuxtla Gutierrez, Chiapas
Tel: +52 961 222 92, Fax: +52 961 249 24

Universidad Autónoma de Chihuahua, Facultad de Medicina [182]

Avenida Colon y Rosales S/N, Chihuahua, Chih. 31350
Tel: +52 14 152 059, Fax: +52 14 152 543

Universidad Autónoma de Ciudad Juárez, Facultad de Medicina [183]

Anillo Envolvente del PRONAF y Estocolmo, Ciudad Juarez, Chih. 32310
Tel: +52 16 88 18 00, Fax: +52 16 88 18 11

Universidad Autónoma de Coahuila, Unidad Saltillo, Facultad de Medicina [184]

Francisco Murguia Sur Num. 205, Saltillo, Coahuila 25000
Tel: +52 84 128 095, Fax: +52 84 128 095

Universidad Autónoma de Coahuila, Unidad Torreon, Facultad de Medicina [185]

Avenida Morelos 900 Oriente, Torreon Cuahuila 27000
Tel: +52 17 137 044, Fax: +52 17 136 783

Universidad Autónoma de Guadalajara, Facultad de Medicina [186]

Hospital Dr. Angel Leaño, Km. 5 Carretera a Tesistán, Guadalajara, Jalisco 44100
Tel: +52 3 834 3968, Fax: +52 3 641 9513

Universidad Autónoma de Nayarit, Escuela de Medicina [187]

Avenida de la Cultura, Tepic, Nayarit 63190
Tel: +52 32 118 817, Fax: +52 32 118 800

Universidad Autónoma de Nuevo Leon, Facultad de Medicina [188]

Hospital Universitario "Dr. José E. Gonzales", Av. Francisco I Madero al Poniente y
Gonzalitos, Monterrey, N.L. 64460
Tel: +52 83 294 153, Fax: +52 83 485 477

Universidad Autónoma de Querétaro, Escuela de Medicina [189]

Clavel No. 200, Fracc. Prado de la Capilla, Querétaro, Qro. 76170
Tel: +52 42 161 414, Fax: +52 42 161 087

Universidad Autónoma de San Luis Potosí, Facultad de Medicina
Avenida Venustiano Carranza Num. 2405, San Luis Potosi, S.L.P. 78210
Tel: +52 48 262 350, Fax: +52 48 262 352

Universidad Autónoma de Sinaloa, Escuela de Medicina
U. Universitaria Obregon y Josefa Ortiz,
Col. Tierra Blanca, Culiacan, Sin. 80030
Tel: +52 67 150 338, Fax: +52 67 150 338

Universidad Autónoma de Tamaulipas, Unidad Tampico, Facultad de Medicina
Centro Universitario Tampico Madero, Tampico, Tamps. 89339
Tel: +52 12 270 576, Fax: +52 12 270 586

Universidad Autónoma de Yucatán, Facultad de Medicina
Avenida Itzaez Num. 498, Mérida, Yuc. 97000
Tel: +52 99 240 554, Fax: +52 99 233 297

Universidad Autónoma de Zacatecas, Facultad de Medicina
Carretera a la Bufa S/N, Zacatecas, Zac. 98000
Tel: +52 492 210 56, Fax: +52 492 246 10

Universidad Autónoma del Estado de Hidalgo, Instituto de Ciencias de la Salud
Dr. Eliseo Ramirez Ulloa Num. 400, col. Doctores, Pachuca de Soto Hidalgo 42090
Tel: +52 771 720 00 ext. 4510, Fax: +52 771 720 00 ext. 4510

Universidad Autónoma del Estado de Morelos, Escuela de Medicina
Avenida Universidad 1001, Colonia Chamilpa, Cuernavaca, Mor. 62210
Tel: +52 73 297 048, Fax: +52 73 297 098

Universidad Autónoma del Estado del México, Facultad de Medicina
Paseo Tollocan y Jesus Carranza S/N, Toluca, Edo. de 50180
Tel: +52 72 173 552, Fax: +52 72 174 831

Universidad Autónoma Metropolitana, Unidad Xochimilco, Carrera de Medicina
Calz. Del Hueso 1110 y Canal Nacional,
Col. Villa Quietud, Coyoacan, México, D.F. 04960
Tel: +52 5 483 7200, Fax: +52 5 483 7200

Universidad de Colima, Facultad de Medicina
Avenida Universidad Num. 333, Colima, Col. 28040
Tel: +52 331 610 99, Fax: +52 331 202 12

Universidad de Guadalajara, Carrera de Medicina
Centro Médico de Occidente, Colonia Independencia,
Guadalajara, Jalisco 44340
Tel: +52 3 617 5022, Fax: +52 3 617 5506

Universidad de Guanajuato, Facultad de Medicina de León
20 de Enero Num. 929, Col. Obregon, Leon, CP 37320
Tel: +52 47 148 455, Fax: +52 47 142 522

Universidad de Montemorelos, Carrera de Medicina
Avenida Libertad Poniente No. 1300, Montemorelos, N.L. 67500
Tel: +52 826 335 10, Fax: +52 826 334 19

Universidad de Monterrey, Division de Ciencias Sociales y de la Salud
Avenida I. Morones Prieto 4500 Poniente,
San Pedro Garza Garcia, N.L. 66238
Tel: +52 8 124 1265, Fax: +52 8 124 1271

Universidad del Noreste, Escuela de Medicina
Prolongación Avenida Hidalgo 6315, Colonia Nuevo Aeropuerto
Tampico, Tam. 89337
Tel: +52 833 228 1117, Fax: +52 833 2281117

Universidad del Ejército y Fuerza Aérea, Escuela Médico Militar
Anillo Periferico y Batallo de Celaya,
Col. Lomas de Sotelo, México, D.F. 11649
Tel: +52 5 520 2056, Fax: +52 5 520 2121

Universidad Juárez Autónoma de Tabasco, Carrera de Medicina
Av. Gregorio Mendez No. 2838-A, Colonia Tamulté, Villa Hermosa, Tab. 86150
Tel: +52 93 540 292, Fax: +52 93 511 105

Universidad Juarez del Estado de Durango, Unidad Durango, Facultad de Medicina
Avenida Universidad y Fanny Anitua, Durango, Dgo. 34000
Tel: +52 18 121 779, Fax: +52 18 130 527

Universidad Juarez del Estado de Durango, Unidad Gomez Palacio, Facultad de
Medicina
Av. La Salle y Calzada Sixto Ugalde, Col. Revolucion, Gomez Palacio, Dgo. 35050
Tel: +52 17 146 476, Fax: +52 146 476

Universidad La Salle, Facultad Mexicana de Medicina
Fuentes Num. 31, Tlalpan, México, D.F. 14000
Tel: +52 5 606 2657, Fax: +52 5 606 3157

Universidad México Americana del Norte, Escuela de Medicina
Guerrero y Plutarco Elias Calles 1317, Colonia Del Prado
Delegacion Benito Juarez, Ciudad Reynosa, Tamps. 88560
Tel: +52 89 222 086, Fax: +52 89 228 568

Universidad Michoacana de San Nicolás de Hidalgo, Facultad de Medicina
Morelia, Mich. 58000
Tel: +52 43 128 239, Fax: +52 43 120 014

Universidad Nacional Autónoma de México (UNAM) México City
Tel: +52 5 292 2377, Fax: +52 5 292 2377 ext. 110

Universidad Nacional Autónoma de México, Facultad de Medicina
Edificio "B" Primer Piso, Circuito Escolar Interior,
Ciudad Universitaria, México, D.F. 04510
Tel: +52 5 616 1162, Fax: +52 5 616 1616

Universidad Nacional Autónoma de México (Iztacala), Escuela Nacional de Estudios
Profesionales Iztacala
Avenida de Los Barrios S/N, Los Reyes, Apdo 314, Tlalnepantla 54090
Tel: +52 5 623 1148, Fax: +52 5 623 1218

Universidad Nacional Autónoma de México (Zaragoza), Facultad de Estudios
Superiores Zaragoza, Carrera de Medicina
Jose C. Bonilla Num. 66, Colonia Ejercito de Ote, Iztapalapa,
México, D.F. 09230
Tel: +52 5 623 0646, Fax: +52 5 623 0657

Universidad Popular Autónoma del Estado de Puebla, Facultad de Medicina
Calle 21 Sur Num. 1103, Colonia Santiago, Puebla, Pue. 72160
Tel: +52 22 299 499 ext. 586, Fax: +52 22 299 499 ext. 526

Universidad Regional del Sureste, Escuela de Medicina y Cirugia
Prolongacion 20 de Noviembre S/N, Col. Miguel Aleman, Oaxaca de Juárez, Oax.
68120
Tel: +52 951 41 410, Fax: +52 951 46 318

Universidad Valle del Bravo, Facultad de Medicina
Calle Septima y Rio Mante S/N, Colonia Prolongacion Longoria, Ciudad Reynosa,
Tamps. 88700
Tel: +52 89 234 722, Fax: +52 89 239 447

Universidad Veracruzana, Unidad Ciudad Mendoza, Facultad de Medicina
Hidalgo Carrillo Puerto, Ciudad Mendoza, Ver. 94740
Tel: +52 272 63 309, Fax: +52 272 71 209

Universidad Veracruzana, Unidad Minatitlán, Facultad de Medicina
>   Atenas y Managua, Col. Nueva Minatitlán, Minatitlán, Ver. 96760
>   Tel: +52 922 12 122, Fax: +52 922 12 123

Universidad Veracruzana, Unidad Poza Rica, Facultad de Medicina
>   Boulevard Lázaro Cárdenas 801, Colonia Morelos, Poza Rica, Ver. 93340
>   Tel: +52 782 25 614, Fax: +52 782 21 241

Universidad Veracruzana, Unidad Veracruz, Facultad de Medicina
>   Iturbide y Carmen Serdán S/N, Veracruz, Ver. 91900
>   Tel: +52 29 324 959, Fax: +52 29 325 534

Universidad Veracruzana, Unidad Xalapa, Facultad de Medicina
>   Odontologos y Médicos S/N, Unidad del Bonque Pensiones Xalapa, Ver. 91010
>   Tel: +52 28 153 443, Fax: +52 28 153 443

Appendix H: Dental Specialists

NAME & ADDRESS	STUDIES & CERTIFICATIONS	LANGUAGES
Algazi de Mekler, Julieta Ave. de las Fuentes 41A Desp. 304, Col. Tecamachalco Tel.: 5589-9124/9166 Specialty: Endodontist	Universidad Autonoma de Mexico; Institute of Endometaendodontics; Member of Association of Endodontists, D.F.	English Spanish French Hebrew
Booth, Belinda Olivera Av. De la Republica (Juarez) 135, Interior 10 Col. Tabacalera, 06030 Tel. 5591-0272 Also available at the following address: Av. San Francisco 16 Col. Del Valle, 03100 Tel. 5543-1759; 10:00-13:00 (or appointment)	UNAM (Oral Surgeon)	English Spanish
Castillo Mendez, Ana Luisa Telchac 301 esq. Tecal Col. Jardines del Ajusco Tel.: 5645-6254 Specialty: Endodontist	University of Mexico	English Spanish
Cornish, Charles K. Felix Berenguer No. 106-401 Col. Lomas Virreyes, 11000 Mexico, D. F. Tel: 5540-2946 & 5540-2948 Fax: 5540-7543 Specialty: General & Restorative Dentistry	University of California	English Spanish
Fuentes Martinez, Jorge Luz Savinon 727, Col. Del Valle 03100 Mexico D.F Tel.: 5523-3615 & 5669-3435 Emergency: 5227-7979 PIN 5589510 Web site address: www.drjorgefuentes.com E-mail address: info@drjorgefuentes.com Specialty: General & Restorative Dentistry	UNAM, Facultad de Odontologia	English Spanish

Gutverg Rosenblum, David S. Presidente Masaryk 191-901 Colonia Polanco 11570 Mexico D.F Tel.: 5282-0320/0322 Fax:5282-0321 Specialty: Periodontal, Implants	Technological University of Mexico; University of Southern California	English Spanish
Hernandez Vargas, Hugo Taine 249-603-4, Col. Polanco 11570 Mexico, D.F. Tel. & Fax: 5531-81-14 Specialty: Dental Surgery	Universidad Latinoamericana	English Spanish
Justus, Roberto Ejercito Nacional No. 530-502 Col. Polanco 11560 Mexico, D.F. Tel.: 5545-7170 & 5531-8466 Fax: 5531-4845 Specialty: Orthodontists	U. of Washington; Seattle, Wa. U. of California	English Spanish German Hungarian
Justus, Yolanda Ejercito Nacional No. 530-501 Col. Polanco 11560 Mexico, D. F. Tel.: 5531-8466 / 5545-7170 Fax: 5531-4847 Specialty: Endodontist (Root Canal, etc.)	U. of Washington; Seattle, Wa. U. of California	English Spanish
Kogan, Enrique Homero 136-3rd floor Col. Polanco C.P. 11570 Tel.: 5545-9872 / 5531-3806 Fax: 5545-5206 Specialty: General & Restorative Dentistry	Technological University of Mexico; University of Missouri-Kansas City	English Spanish
Konstat, Manuel Palmas 735-1201, Col. Lomas Tel.: 5202-7883 / 5202-7835 Specialty: Children's Dentistry	Tufts University School of Dentistry; American Academy of Pedodontics	English Spanish German Yiddish Hebrew

Naffah Kamel, Joseph Bosques de Duraznos 65-709 Col. Bosques de las Lomas Tel.: 5596-5447 / 5251-4206 Fax : 5251-0511 Specialty: Children's Odontologist.	Metropolitan Autonomous University, Mexico City Western Reserve University Cleveland, Ohio	English Spanish Portuguese French Arabic
Nestel, Enrique Homero 1804-1001, Col. Polanco 11570 Mexico, D.F. Tel.: 5395-3162 Fax : 5395-3138 Specialty: Orthodontist	University of Washington Unitec in Mexico	English Spanish Hebrew Yiddish
Nischli Gasman, Arie Paseo de las Palmas 830-201 Col. Lomas de Chapultepec 11000 Mexico D.F. Tel. 5540-0411, 5540-4900 Specialty: Orthodontist	Technological University of Mexico Boston University Member: American Association of Orthodontists	Spanish English Italian French Hebrew
Nurko, Flora Temistocles 56-PB Col. Polanco Tel.: 5281-2043 / 5280-7248 Specialty: Fixed prostheses	Children's Hospital of Pennsylvania; Universidad Autonoma de Mexico	English Spanish
Ovadia A., Eduardo Ave. de las Fuentes 41A-901 Col. Tecamachalco C.P. 53950 Tel: 5294- 0873 Specialty: Children's Dentistry	University of Southern California with Children's Hospital of Los Angeles	English Spanish
Ovadia, Victor Ave. de las Fuentes 41A-303 Col. Tecamachalco Tel.:5294-1031 / 5294-5122 / 0859 Specialty: Children's Dentistry	Universidad Tecnologica de Mexico Boston University School of Dentistry	English Spanish
Oynick V., Jose Prado Sur 480, Col. Lomas Tel.: 5520-8567 & 5540-3856 Specialty: Endodontics	Universidad Autonoma de Mexico	English Spanish French

Oynick, Tamara Prado Sur 480 P.B., Col. Lomas de Chapultepec, C.P. 11560 Tel.: 5540-3856 & 5520-8567 Specialty: Endodontics	Universidad Tecnologica de Mexico	English Spanish French
Ramos-Tercero, Jose A. Providencia 1218 - PB Col. del Valle 03100 Mexico, D.F. Tel. 5559-95-99 Specialty: Pediatric Dentistry	Universidad Tecnologica de Mexico, University of Texas Health Science at San Antonio, Texas	English Spanish
Romanowsky, Jaime H. 655 Prado Norte, Suite 302 Col. Lomas de Chapultepec Tel.: 5540-6815 / 5540-6817 / 5540-6816 / 5540-3166 Specialty: General & Restorative Dentistry	Technological University of Mexico; Harvard School of Dental Medicine	English Spanish Hebrew German
Rotberg, Saul B. Ejercito Nacional 650-104 Col. Polanco 11560 – Mexico, D.F. Tel.: 5531-8839/9619, 5545-4515 Fax : 5545-0063 Specialty: Orthodontia	Technological University of Mexico; Tufts University Member of the American Orthodontist Association	English Spanish Hebrew
Rotberg, Roberto B. Ejercito Nacional 650-104 Col. Polanco 11560 – Mexico, D.F. Tel.: 5531-8839 / 5531-9619 / 5545-4515 Specialty: Orthodontia	Technological University of Mexico; Tufts University Member of the American Orthodontist Association	English Spanish Hebrew
Pinedo Rodriguez, Oscar Torres Adalid 205 – 302 Col. Del Valle 03100 Mexico, D.F. Tel.: 5523-73-87 / 5543-23-55 Specialty: General Orthodontia	Facultad de Odontologia, UNAM Centro de Investigacion y Especializacion en Rehabilitacion Oral, A.C.	English Spanish

Rubinstein, Jaime M. Bosques de Duraznos 65-1007-A Tel.: 5251-8121 Fax : 5251-9299 Specialty: Pediatric Dentistry	Universidad Autonoma de Mexico; University of Illinois	English Spanish Hebrew Yiddish
Sakar Allende, Alfredo Presa Sanalona No. 8 Col. Irrigacion 11520 – Mexico, D. F. Tel.: 5557-1145 / 5557-1138 / 5557-0812. Emergency 5227- 7979 Fax: 5557-8147 Specialty: Prosthodontics, Restorative Dentistry & Implants.	University of Texas Health Science Center Dental Branch Houston	English Spanish
Sanchez Woodworth, Robert Bosque de Durazno 69-303 Bosques de Las Lomas Tel.: 5596-1244 / 5596-3722 / 5596-3245 Fax : 5596-3414 Specialty: Orthodontia	Loyola University; St. Louis University; Mexican Association of Orthodontists	English Spanish French
Tobias, Mario Palmas 745-201, Col. Lomas Tel.: 5540-2486 & 5520-0269 Specialty: Children's Dentistry	Tufts University; Children's Hospital, Pennsylvania	English Spanish Yiddish, Hebrew French
Ugalde, Francisco Javier Hospital Español Ejercito Nacional 613 Col. Polanco Tel: 5531-9529, 5531-9530, 5531-9531 e-mail: francisco_javieru@hotmail.com Specialty: Orthodontia	Universidad Tecnologica de Mexico; M.S. in Orthodontics Member of the Mexico City Orthodontics Association	Spanish English
Zfaz, Victor P.Palmas-830-101. Col. Lomas de Chapultepec Tel.: 5540-6767 / 5540-6655 / 5540-0919 Specialty: General & Restorative Dentistry	UNAM Dental School; Univ. of Jerusalem, Israel American Dental Association	English Spanish Yiddish

Appendix I: The Insurance Grid

This grid is designed to help you sort through the many factors you may want to consider when deciding what types of coverage or benefits you may need.

Type of Insurance or Health-Related Benefit	Typically Designed to Cover This	Things You Should Know About It
Employee Health Insurance (or COBRA from a former employer in the USA)	Covers healthcare costs incurred in home country only. Typically, it will not provide coverage—or only limited coverage—while traveling. May not provide any benefits outside of your home country at all.	Some policies provide only emergency coverage or coverage for only a limited number of days. Check with your employer. You will have to file any claims yourself and be reimbursed for any covered expenses. If you don't have other coverage, you may have to pay all medical expenses out of pocket. Mexico does not have reciprocal agreements with other countries, so you must obtain other coverage if you are covered under a government program.
Preventative Healthcare Benefits	Coverage for routine checkups designed to detect medical conditions early. Often a part of Employee Health Insurance.	Traditional domestic U.S. health insurance plans may have wellness (health checkup) benefits but the member usually cannot take advantage of these benefits in Mexico. Consider a Mexican HMO-type program affiliated with a local medical practice or group. [See Private Clinic Programs & Discount Medical Memberships below]
Government health programs in Canada, European nations, etc.	These provide coverage in your home country or countries with reciprocal agreements with your home country. These do NOT apply to Mexico. There are no mutual agreements with Mexico.	Traditional domestic U.S. health insurance plans may have wellness (health checkup) benefits but the member usually cannot take advantage of these benefits in Mexico. Consider a Mexican HMO-type program affiliated with a local medical practice or group. [See Private Clinic Programs & Discount Medical Memberships below]

Short Term International Health Plans (Traveler's Insurance, Traveler's Medical Plans)	Coverage for up to three years outside home country. Can cover costs of hospital and doctors, medicine, local and air ambulance, reunion of family members, and offer 24-hour-a- day, seven days a week support.	You will be required to show a credit card and/or proof of insurance before being treated in most private hospitals in Mexico. These policies are ideal for visitors staying a few weeks or months, students and professionals. For longer stays, consider International Major Medical Plans. Traveler's insurance must be obtained in your home country before arriving in Mexico, although it can be obtained online.
Travel Assistance Benefits	Typically these are additional services that are added to Traveler's Insurance.	Beyond medical and hospital coverage, you may find that communication with your family, finding a doctor and communications in general become more complex in an emergency. Travel assistance benefits offer support in English when and where you need it.
International Major Medical Plans	Coverage in Europe and Latin America. Can cover costs of hospital and doctors, medicine, local and air ambulance, reunion of family members, and offer 24-hour-a-day, seven days a week support.	You will be required to show a credit card and/or proof of insurance before being treated in most private hospitals in Mexico. Can include home country coverage or even worldwide coverage. You can typically choose policy limits between $50,000-8 million USD. Will pay for private hospital care.
Bi-National Insurance	These are medical plans that cover individuals or families on either side of the USA/Mexican border.	These policies are typically only available in border regions, particularly in California and are often preferred by people who want to receive medical care in Mexico with Spanish-speaking physicians, but who live and/or work in the USA. Coverage is typically limited to border cities.
Mexican Health Insurance	Widely available and accepted medical and/or hospital benefits for a monthly premium. May be obtained through employment in Mexico. Can be purchased through brokers, banks and directly through carriers.	Coverage and premiums vary and typically coverage is only available in Mexico. Policies are typically in Spanish. May have limits, exclusions on pre-existing conditions, etc.

Medicare & Medicaid	Provides healthcare benefits for US citizens age 65 or over or low-income individuals or families within the USA only. The hospital insurance part of Medicare is available to you if you return to the United States. No monthly premium is withheld from your benefit payment for this protection. Other medical care requires premium payment.	It is not always possible to get a ticket and fly back to your home country in the case of a health emergency or accident. Consider Evacuation Insurance to supplement Medicare. Also, you may require or prefer local hospitalization. Consider IMSS if you have an temporary or permanent resident visa or an International Major Medical Plan.
IMSS (Instituto Mexicano del Seguro Social)	A Mexican government program that covers all working Mexicans on a mandatory basis and others on a voluntary basis. Offers full coverage including medical and hospital care and pharmaceuticals at a low annual premium.	Only expats with a temporary or permanent resident visa qualify. Takes up to 2 years for full coverage. Pre-existing conditions are not covered. Quality varies regionally. Enrollment is a fairly complex process. A primary-care physician makes all referrals to specialists (similar to an HMO). Runs its own hospital system.
Private Clinic Programs & Discount Medical Memberships	These are private, Mexican- based membership programs that offer a range of health benefits, wellness and entertainment, at the national level through a wide range of providers (doctors, specialists, laboratories, pharmacies, hospitals, restaurants, gyms, nutrition and more) with preferential prices, discounts or certificates.	While the program benefits will vary, they can include phone consultations, home visits, ambulance, discounted hospitalization, dental and vision care, etc. They do not offer full hospitalization benefits and function more like the Preventative Healthcare Benefits of a HMO or PPO, but without major medical or hospital coverage.
Medical Evacuation Insurance	Provides air and ground transportation with skilled medical care and other medical assistance to move the ill or injured from one part of the world to another in the event of a medical emergency. Benefits vary, however the best will take you to hospital of your choice.	A medically necessary air ambulance can cost $30,000 USD or more. Some medical air evacuation policies have a 90-day waiting period on pre- existing medical conditions. Some cover any hospitalization, while others are more restrictive. Most do not cover medical expenses. May help an expat take advantage of benefits such as Medicare in their home country when they become seriously ill in Mexico.
Long Term Care Insurance	Can often be used to pay the medical and other care expenses in Mexico for someone who is chronically ill.	You will want to make certain that your plan will pay benefits for care in Mexico and what the claims process would be.

Elective Surgery	Private financing	Most elective surgery is excluded from coverage under regular health insurance plans. This can include cosmetic surgeries, "experimental" procedures and surgeries that may be life-enhancing or even life saving for the individual such as bariatric surgery for obesity.
Employer International Group Medical plans	Provides group coverage for 2 or more people who work together.	Typically covers Canada, Mexico and the USA, but can be configured to cover Mexico only for savings.
International Life Insurance	Provides cash to your family or business partners after you die	With Latin America-based policies, the insurer would buy dollars to pay the death benefit or pay it in local currency.
Disability Income Protection	Provides income if you should suffer a disability.	This is often an "add on" benefit of some life insurance policies.
Foreign Medical Program for Disabled US Veterans	A USA program that provides full medical coverage in foreign countries in addition to other benefits for disabled veterans.	Medical bills will either need to be produced in English or translated by the VA. The VA must certify your disability. You will be reimbursed by check.
Vehicle Insurance for Mexico	Your vehicle insurance should provide liability coverage to pay medical costs for injured passengers in your car or those in any other vehicles involved in addition to collision, legal representation and bail-bond coverage if you are arrested.	Your car insurance from outside of Mexico will not provide coverage in Mexico. If you are going to drive in Mexico it is essential that your vehicle be adequately insured. You will be held immediately responsible for all expenses for any accident you are involved in and you cannot rely on other drivers to have insurance.
High Risk Activities Insurance	Some sports or activities are excluded from benefits under regular Traveler's Insurance or International Major Medical Plans.	If you plan to go gliding, hang-gliding, paragliding, rock climbing, parachuting, shark diving or other high risk or hazardous activity, you will probably need special coverage and/or to pay an additional premium. Check with your carrier. Do not assume you are covered.

Appendix J: Retirement Communities, Assisted Living & Nursing Care

http://abbeyfield-ajijic.org/

http://casacieneguita-assisted-living.com/

http://www.lacasanostra.com.mx/

http://lakesidecare.com/

http://lasgardenias.com.mx/

http://www.lavalentinarc.com/

http://losarroyosverdes.com/

http://mexicoassistedliving.com/

http://seniorcareinmexico.com/

http://seniorslivingmexico.com/

http://www.abbeyfield-ajijic.org/

http://www.aliciaconvalescent.com/

http://www.cielitolindoassistedliving.com/

http://www.dondemiraelsol.com/

http://www.kuunbeek.com/

http://www.laamada.com/

http://www.lamoralejaresidencial.com/Inicio.html

http://www.lapueblita.com/

http://www.latierra-prometida.com/

http://www.lumaliving.com/

http://www.quintalegre.com.mx/

http://www.residencialasmagnolias.org.mx/home.asp

http://www.sageatoasisofhope.com/en/

http://www.seniorliving.com.mx/

http://www.serenaseniorcare.com/

http://www.tetexopa.com/

http://www.ventanasresidences.com/

http://www.villazul.com.mx/index.php

http://yucatancountry.com/

Appendix K: Mexico's Palliative Care Law

DECRETO por el que se reforma y adiciona la Ley General de Salud en Materia de Cuidados Paliativos.

Al margen un sello con el Escudo Nacional, que dice: Estados Unidos Mexicanos.- Presidencia de la República.

FELIPE DE JESÚS CALDERÓN HINOJOSA, Presidente de los Estados Unidos Mexicanos, a sus habitantes sabed:

Que el Honorable Congreso de la Unión, se ha servido dirigirme el siguiente

DECRETO

"EL CONGRESO GENERAL DE LOS ESTADOS UNIDOS MEXICANOS, DECRETA:

**SE REFORMA Y ADICIONA LA LEY GENERAL DE SALUD EN
MATERIA DE CUIDADOS PALIATIVOS.**

Artículo Primero. Se reforma la fracción I del inciso B del artículo 13; la fracción III del artículo 27; el artículo 59; la fracción III del artículo 112, y el artículo 421 bis; se adiciona la fracción XXX recorriéndose las demás al artículo 3o., y la fracción IV al artículo 33, todos de la Ley General de Salud, para quedar como sigue:

Artículo 3o. ...

I. a XXVIII Bis. ...

XXIX. La sanidad internacional;

XXX. El tratamiento integral del dolor, y

XXXI. ...

Artículo 13. La competencia entre la Federación y las entidades federativas en materia de salubridad general quedará distribuida conforme a lo siguiente:

A. ...

I. a X. ...

B. Corresponde a los gobiernos de las entidades federativas, en materia de salubridad general, como autoridades locales y dentro de sus respectivas jurisdicciones territoriales:

I. Organizar, operar, supervisar y evaluar la prestación de los servicios de salubridad general a que se refieren las fracciones II, IV, V, VI, VII, VIII, IX, X, XI, XII, XIII, XIV, XV, XVI, XVII, XVIII, XIX, XX, XXI, XXII, XXVIII Bis y XXX del artículo 3o. de esta Ley, de conformidad con las disposiciones aplicables;

II. a VII. ...

Artículo 27. ... I. y

II. ...

III. La atención médica integral, que comprende actividades preventivas, curativas, paliativas y de rehabilitación, incluyendo la atención de urgencias;

IV. a X. ...

Artículo 33. Las actividades de atención médica son: I. ...

II. Curativas, que tienen como fin efectuar un diagnóstico temprano y proporcionar tratamiento oportuno; III.

De rehabilitación, que incluyen acciones tendientes a corregir las invalideces físicas o mentales, y

IV. Paliativas, que incluyen el cuidado integral para preservar la calidad de vida del paciente, a través de la prevención, tratamiento y control del dolor, y otros síntomas físicos y emocionales por parte de un equipo profesional multidisciplinario.

Artículo 59. Las dependencias y entidades del sector salud y los gobiernos de las entidades federativas, promoverán y apoyarán la constitución de grupos, asociaciones y demás instituciones que tengan por objeto participar organizadamente en los programas de promoción y mejoramiento de la salud individual o colectiva, así como en los de prevención de enfermedades y accidentes, y de prevención de invalidez y de rehabilitación de inválidos, así como en los cuidados paliativos.

Artículo 112. La educación para la salud tiene por objeto: I. y

II. ...

III. Orientar y capacitar a la población preferentemente en materia de nutrición, salud mental, salud bucal, educación sexual, planificación familiar, cuidados paliativos, riesgos de automedicación, prevención de fármacodependencia, salud ocupacional, salud visual, salud auditiva, uso adecuado de los servicios de salud, prevención de accidentes, prevención y rehabilitación de la invalidez y detección oportuna de enfermedades.

Artículo 421 bis. Se sancionará con multa equivalente de doce mil hasta dieciséis mil veces el salario mínimo general diario vigente en la zona económica de que se trate, la violación de las disposiciones contenidas en los artículos 100, 122, 126, 146, 166 Bis 19, 166 Bis 20, 205, 235, 254, 264, 281, 289, 293, 298, 325, 327 y 333 de esta Ley.

Artículo Segundo. Se crea un Título Octavo Bis denominado "De los Cuidados Paliativos a los Enfermos en Situación Terminal".

TITULO OCTAVO BIS

De los Cuidados Paliativos a los Enfermos en Situación Terminal

CAPÍTULO I Disposiciones

Comunes

Artículo 166 Bis. El presente título tiene por objeto:

I.   Salvaguardar la dignidad de los enfermos en situación terminal, para garantizar una vida de calidad a través de los cuidados y atenciones médicas, necesarios para ello;

II. Garantizar una muerte natural en condiciones dignas a los enfermos en situación terminal;

III. Establecer y garantizar los derechos del enfermo en situación terminal en relación con su tratamiento;

IV. Dar a conocer los límites entre el tratamiento curativo y el paliativo;

V.   Determinar los medios ordinarios y extraordinarios en los tratamientos; y

VI. Establecer los límites entre la defensa de la vida del enfermo en situación terminal y la obstinación terapéutica.

Artículo 166 Bis 1. Para los efectos de este Título, se entenderá por:

I. Enfermedad en estado terminal. A todo padecimiento reconocido, irreversible, progresivo e incurable que se encuentra en estado avanzado y cuyo pronóstico de vida para el paciente sea menor a 6 meses;

II. Cuidados básicos. La higiene, alimentación e hidratación, y en su caso el manejo de la vía aérea permeable;

III. Cuidados Paliativos. Es el cuidado activo y total de aquéllas enfermedades que no responden a tratamiento curativo. El control del dolor, y de otros síntomas, así como la atención de aspectos psicológicos, sociales y espirituales;

IV. Enfermo en situación terminal. Es la persona que tiene una enfermedad incurable e irreversible y que tiene un pronóstico de vida inferior a seis meses;

V. Obstinación terapéutica. La adopción de medidas desproporcionadas o inútiles con el objeto de alargar la vida en situación de agonía;

VI. Medios extraordinarios. Los que constituyen una carga demasiado grave para el enfermo y cuyo perjuicio es mayor que los beneficios; en cuyo caso, se podrán valorar estos medios en comparación al tipo de terapia, el grado de dificultad y de riesgo que comporta, los gastos necesarios y las posibilidades de aplicación respecto del resultado que se puede esperar de todo ello;

VII. Medios ordinarios. Los que son útiles para conservar la vida del enfermo en situación terminal o para curarlo y que no constituyen, para él una carga grave o desproporcionada a los beneficios que se pueden obtener;

VIII. Muerte natural. El proceso de fallecimiento natural de un enfermo en situación terminal, contando con asistencia física, psicológica y en su caso, espiritual; y

IX. Tratamiento del dolor. Todas aquellas medidas proporcionadas por profesionales de la salud, orientadas a reducir los sufrimientos físico y emocional producto de una enfermedad terminal, destinadas a mejorar la calidad de vida.

Artículo 166 Bis 2. Corresponde al Sistema Nacional de Salud garantizar el pleno, libre e informado ejercicio de los derechos que señalan esta Ley y demás ordenamientos aplicables, a los enfermos en situación terminal.

CAPÍTULO II

De los Derechos de los Enfermos en Situación Terminal

Artículo 166 Bis 3. Los pacientes enfermos en situación terminal tienen los siguientes derechos: I. Recibir atención médica integral;

II. Ingresar a las instituciones de salud cuando requiera atención médica;

III. Dejar voluntariamente la institución de salud en que esté hospitalizado, de conformidad a las disposiciones aplicables;

IV. Recibir un trato digno, respetuoso y profesional procurando preservar su calidad de vida;

V. Recibir información clara, oportuna y suficiente sobre las condiciones y efectos de su enfermedad y los tipos de tratamientos por los cuales puede optar según la enfermedad que padezca;

VI. Dar su consentimiento informado por escrito para la aplicación o no de tratamientos, medicamentos y cuidados paliativos adecuados a su enfermedad, necesidades y calidad de vida;

VII. Solicitar al médico que le administre medicamentos que mitiguen el dolor;

VIII. Renunciar, abandonar o negarse en cualquier momento a recibir o continuar el tratamiento que considere extraordinario;

IX. Optar por recibir los cuidados paliativos en un domicilio particular;

X. Designar, a algún familiar, representante legal o a una persona de su confianza, para el caso de que, con el avance de la enfermedad, esté impedido a expresar su voluntad, lo haga en su representación;

XI. A recibir los servicios espirituales, cuando lo solicite él, su familia, representante legal o persona de su confianza; y

XII. Los demás que las leyes señalen.

Artículo 166 Bis 4. Toda persona mayor de edad, en pleno uso de sus facultades mentales, puede, en cualquier momento e independientemente de su estado de salud, expresar su voluntad por escrito ante dos testigos, de recibir o no cualquier tratamiento, en caso de que llegase a padecer una enfermedad y estar en situación terminal y no le sea posible manifestar dicha voluntad. Dicho documento podrá ser revocado en cualquier momento.

Para que sea válida la disposición de voluntad referida en el párrafo anterior, deberá apegarse a lo dispuesto en la presente Ley y demás disposiciones aplicables.

Artículo 166 Bis 5. El paciente en situación terminal, mayor de edad y en pleno uso de sus facultades mentales, tiene derecho a la suspensión voluntaria del tratamiento curativo y como consecuencia al inicio de tratamiento estrictamente paliativo en la forma y términos previstos en esta Ley.

Artículo 166 Bis 6. La suspensión voluntaria del tratamiento curativo supone la cancelación de todo medicamento que busque contrarrestar la enfermedad terminal del paciente y el inicio de tratamientos enfocados de manera exclusiva a la disminución del dolor o malestar del paciente.

En este caso, el médico especialista en el padecimiento del paciente terminal interrumpe, suspende o no inicia el tratamiento, la administración de medicamentos, el uso de instrumentos o cualquier procedimiento que contribuya a la prolongación de la vida del paciente en situación terminal dejando que su padecimiento evolucione naturalmente.

Artículo 166 Bis 7. El paciente en situación terminal que esté recibiendo los cuidados paliativos, podrá solicitar recibir nuevamente el tratamiento curativo, ratificando su decisión por escrito ante el personal médico correspondiente.

Artículo 166 Bis 8. Si el enfermo en situación terminal es menor de edad, o se encuentra incapacitado para expresar su voluntad, las decisiones derivadas de los derechos señalados en este título, serán asumidos por los padres o el tutor y a falta de estos por su representante legal, persona de su confianza mayor de edad o juez de conformidad con las disposiciones aplicables.

Artículo 166 Bis 9. Los cuidados paliativos se proporcionarán desde el momento en que se diagnostica el estado terminal de la enfermedad, por el médico especialista.

Artículo 166 Bis 10. Los familiares del enfermo en situación terminal tienen la obligación de respetar la decisión que de manera voluntaria tome el enfermo en los términos de este título.

Artículo 166 Bis 11. En casos de urgencia médica, y que exista incapacidad del enfermo en situación terminal para expresar su consentimiento, y en ausencia de familiares, representante legal, tutor o persona de confianza, la decisión de aplicar un procedimiento médico quirúrgico o tratamiento necesario, será tomada por el médico especialista y/o por el Comité de Bioética de la institución.

Artículo 166 Bis 12. Todos los documentos a que se refiere este título se regirán de acuerdo a lo que se establezca en el reglamento y demás disposiciones aplicables.

CAPÍTULO III

De las Facultades y Obligaciones de las Instituciones de Salud

Artículo 166 Bis 13. Las Instituciones del Sistema Nacional de Salud:

I. Ofrecerán el servicio para la atención debida a los enfermos en situación terminal;

II. Proporcionarán los servicios de orientación, asesoría y seguimiento al enfermo en situación terminal y o sus familiares o persona de confianza en el caso de que los cuidados paliativos se realicen en el domicilio particular;

III. De igual manera, en el caso de que los cuidados paliativos se realicen en el domicilio particular, la Secretaría pondrá en operación una línea telefónica de acceso gratuito para que se le oriente, asesore y dé seguimiento al enfermo en situación terminal o a sus familiares o persona de su confianza;

IV. Proporcionarán los cuidados paliativos correspondientes al tipo y grado de enfermedad, desde el momento del diagnóstico de la enfermedad terminal hasta el último momento;

V. Fomentarán la creación de áreas especializadas que presten atención a los enfermos en situación terminal; y

VI. Garantizarán la capacitación y actualización permanente de los recursos humanos para la salud, en materia de cuidados paliativos y atención a enfermos en situación terminal.

CAPÍTULO IV

De los Derechos, Facultades y Obligaciones de los Médicos y Personal Sanitario

Artículo 166 Bis 14. Los médicos tratantes y el equipo sanitario que preste los cuidados paliativos, para el mejor desempeño de sus servicios, deberán estar debidamente capacitados humana y técnicamente, por instituciones autorizadas para ello.

Artículo 166 Bis 15. Los médicos especialistas en las instituciones de segundo y tercer nivel, tendrán las siguientes obligaciones:

I. Proporcionar toda la información que el paciente requiera, así como la que el médico considere necesaria para que el enfermo en situación terminal pueda tomar una decisión libre e informada sobre su atención, tratamiento y cuidados;

II. Pedir el consentimiento informado del enfermo en situación terminal, por escrito ante dos testigos, para los tratamientos o medidas a tomar respecto de la enfermedad terminal;

III. Informar oportunamente al enfermo en situación terminal, cuando el tratamiento curativo no dé resultados;

IV. Informar al enfermo en situación terminal, sobre las opciones que existan de cuidados paliativos;

V. Respetar la decisión del enfermo en situación terminal en cuanto al tratamiento curativo y cuidados paliativos, una vez que se le haya explicado en términos sencillos las consecuencias de su decisión;

VI. Garantizar que se brinden los cuidados básicos o tratamiento al paciente en todo momento;

VII. Procurar las medidas mínimas necesaria para preservar la calidad de vida de los enfermos en situación terminal;

VIII. Respetar y aplicar todas y cada una de las medidas y procedimientos para los casos que señala esta ley;

IX. Hacer saber al enfermo, de inmediato y antes de su aplicación, si el tratamiento a seguir para aliviar el dolor y los síntomas de su enfermedad tenga como posibles efectos secundarios disminuir el tiempo de vida;

X. Solicitar una segunda opinión a otro médico especialista, cuando su diagnóstico sea una enfermedad terminal; y

XI. Las demás que le señalen ésta y otras leyes.

Artículo 166 Bis 16. Los médicos tratantes podrán suministrar fármacos paliativos a un enfermo en situación terminal, aún cuando con ello se pierda estado de alerta o se acorte la vida del paciente, siempre y cuando se suministren dichos fármacos paliativos con el objeto de aliviar el dolor del paciente.

Podrán hacer uso, de ser necesario de acuerdo con lo estipulado en la presente Ley de analgésicos del grupo de los opioides. En estos casos será necesario el consentimiento del enfermo.

En ningún caso se suministrarán tales fármacos con la finalidad de acortar o terminar la vida del paciente, en tal caso se estará sujeto a las disposiciones penales aplicables.

Artículo 166 Bis 17. Los médicos tratantes, en ningún caso y por ningún motivo implementaran medios extraordinarios al enfermo en situación terminal, sin su consentimiento.

Artículo 166 Bis 18. Para garantizar una vida de calidad y el respeto a la dignidad del enfermo en situación terminal, el personal médico no deberá aplicar tratamientos o medidas consideradas como obstinación terapéutica ni medios extraordinarios.

Artículo 166 Bis 19. El personal médico que deje de proporcionar los cuidados básicos a los enfermos en situación terminal, será sancionado conforme lo establecido por las leyes aplicables.

Artículo 166 Bis 20. El personal médico que, por decisión propia, deje de proporcionar cualquier tratamiento o cuidado sin el consentimiento del enfermo en situación terminal, o en caso que esté impedido para expresar su voluntad, el de su familia o persona de confianza, será sancionado conforme lo establecido por las leyes aplicables.

Artículo 166 Bis 21. Queda prohibida, la práctica de la eutanasia, entendida como homicidio por piedad así como el suicidio asistido conforme lo señala el Código Penal Federal, bajo el amparo de esta ley. En tal caso se estará a lo que señalan las disposiciones penales aplicables.

Transitorios

Artículo Primero.- La Secretaría de Salud deberá emitir los reglamentos y Normas Oficiales Mexicanas que sean necesarios para garantizar el ejercicio de los derechos que concede este Título.

Artículo Segundo.- La Secretaría de Salud tendrá 180 días naturales para expedir el Reglamento respectivo de este Título, contados a partir de la entrada en vigor del presente Decreto.

Artículo Tercero.- El presente Decreto entrará en vigor al día siguiente de su publicación en el Diario Oficial de la Federación.

México, D.F., a 25 de noviembre de 2008.- Dip. **Cesar Horacio Duarte Jaquez**, Presidente.- Sen. **Gustavo Enrique Madero Muñoz**, Presidente.- Dip. **Rosa Elia Romero Guzman**, Secretaria.- Sen. **Ludivina Menchaca Castellanos**, Secretaria.- Rúbricas."

En cumplimiento de lo dispuesto por la fracción I del Artículo 89 de la Constitución Política de los Estados Unidos Mexicanos, y para su debida publicación y observancia, expido el presente Decreto en la Residencia del Poder Ejecutivo Federal, en la Ciudad de México, Distrito Federal, a veintidós de diciembre de dos mil ocho.- **Felipe de Jesús Calderón Hinojosa**.- Rúbrica.- El Secretario de Gobernación, Lic. **Fernando Francisco Gómez Mont Urueta**.- Rúbrica.

Appendix L: Sample Health Care Directive Letter

[This is a Google translation into English. Your letter must be in Spanish. The original Spanish version of this sample letter is published below.]

TO my doctor, hospital or other health care professionals who may be in attendance when I am unable to express my wishes:

When it is determined that my condition is terminal and irreversible and that I'm expected to live less than six months and that I am unable to make informed decisions regarding my care, the following health care directives shall define my care as authorized by *Titulo Octavo de Ley General de Salud,* **a copy of which is attached.**

When I am comatose or otherwise unable to make informed decisions regarding my care, I authorize *[name]* **to make medical decisions on my behalf in addition to my directives listed below. If** *[name]* **is unable to serve, I designate** *[name].*

[Include any of the following example paragraphs or others as you may want and/or as your doctor may recommend: Be sure your directives concur with the law which should be shown where possible. If you include instructions that are beyond the scope of the law, your care giver is not obligated to follow them although he may voluntarily accommodate your wishes.]

I want to receive drugs or other treatments that will keep me comfortable and relieve pain even though this may shorten my life. (Chapter IV, Art 166, Bis16)

I do not want any extraordinary life sustaining measures. This includes being connected to any machines, heart resuscitation and intravenous fluids. (Chapter IV, Art 166, Bis17 and 18)

When practical, I want to receive palliative care in a private home. (Chapter II, Article 166, Bis 3 IX) This decision should be made by my designated representative in consultation with my doctor.

I write this while I am mentally capable of making these decisions. (Chapter II, Art 166, Bis 4)

Date: _____

Patient ___Your Signature_____
Typed name

Witness ___Signature_____
Typed name

Witness ___Signature_____
Typed name

A mi médico, hospital u otros profesionales de la salud que pueden estar presentes cuando no estoy en condiciones de expresar mis deseos:

Cuando se determina que mi condición es terminal e irreversible y que soy una esperanza de vida inferior a seis meses y que soy incapaz de tomar decisiones informadas con respecto a mi cuidado, la atención de la salud directivas siguientes definir mi atención de lo autorizado por el *Titulo Octavo de la Ley General de Salud,* cuya copia se adjunta.

Cuando estoy en estado de coma o no pueda tomar decisiones informadas con respecto a mi cuidado, yo autorizo a *[name]* para tomar decisiones médicas en mi nombre, además de mi directivas que figuran a continuación. Si *[nombre]* es incapaz de servir, designo a *[nombre].*

Deseo recibir medicamentos u otros tratamientos que me mantendrá cómodo y aliviar el dolor, aunque esto puede acortar mi vida. *(Capítulo IV, Art. 166, Bis16)*

No quiero que ninguna de la extraordinaria vida de las medidas de mantenimiento. Esto incluye estar conectado a ninguna máquina, la reanimación del corazón y los líquidos intra-venosos. *(Capítulo IV, Art. 166, Bis 17 y 18)*

Cuando sea posible, quiero recibir los cuidados paliativos en un domicilio particular. *(Capítulo II, artículo 166 Bis 3 IX)* Esta decisión debe ser tomada por mi representante designado en consulta con mi médico.

Escribo esto ahora que estoy mentalmente capaz de tomar estas decisiones. *(Capítulo II, artículo 166, Bis 4)*

Fecha:

Paciente _____

Testigo _____

Testigo _____

Appendix M: Cost Comparisons, USA & Mexico

General Procedures	USA Hospitals	Mexico	Average Savings
Heart			
Angioplasty	$22,500	$11,500	50%
Angiography	$4,800	$1,200	70%
Valve replacement	$ 46,000	$16,000	60%
Bypass surgery	$44,000	$24,000	50%
Open Heart surgery	$64,000	$24,000	66%
Orthopedic			
Knee	$25,000	$10,500	65%
Hip Replacement	$28,000	$12,500	65%
Shoulder Replacement	$24,500	$9,500	75%
Birmingham Resurfacing	$24,000	$12,500	60%

Other Procedures

Cosmetic Procedures	USA Clinic	Cancun, Mexico	Average Savings
Face Lift	$18,000	$4,250	68%
Breast Augmentation	$7,800	$3,800	55%
Tummy Tuck	$8,800	$4,500	50%
Liposuction (per area)	$3,200	$1,150	60%
Rhinoplasty (nose)	$8,000	$3,200	65%
Brow Lift	$7,500	$2,850	70%
Brazilian Buttock	$10,500	$4,950	65%
Neck Lift	$10,000	$4,400	70%
Blepharoplasty (eyelids)	$5,400	$2,950	55%

Dental Procedures	USA Clinic	Monterrey, Mexico	Average Savings
Implants - 6 teeth	$18,500	$3,600	75%
Porcelain crown (6 teeth)	$5,200	$1,600	70%
Bleaching discolored teeth	$250	$50	80%
Dental Veneers (6 teeth)	$6,000	$1,800	75%
Total Dentures	$4,800	$1,600	70%

The following data was gathered by Paul Kurtzweil and his wife of Two Expats Living in Mexico.[190] It is published here with their permission. They compiled the data through personal visit to facilities and providers: hospitals, clinics, doctors' offices, dental offices and laboratories from Tulum to Puerto Morelos. This area tends to have many expats and tends to be more expensive than other parts of Mexico. The prices are given both in Mexican pesos (MXN) and U.S. dollars (USD). The exchange rate used is 18.5 MXN to 1 USD.

Dental

Consultation:	$200 – $500 MXN	[$10.81 – $27.02 USD]
Cleaning + checkup:	$700 – $1700 MXN	[$37.83 – $91.89 USD]
Fill a cavity:	$500 – $800 MXN	[$27.02 – $43.02 USD]
Crown:	$2500 – $7000 MXN	[$135 – $378 USD]
Crown with an implant:	$9000 – $1100 MXN	[$486 – $594 USD]

Dermatologist

Consultation:	$600 – $750 MXN	[$32.43 – $40.54 USD]
Surgery to remove a blemish or mole:	$2000 – $2500 MXN	[$108 – $135 USD]
Surgery to remove skin cancer		
(less than 1 cm):	$7000 – $8000 MXN	[$378 – $432 USD]
(more than 1 cm):	$9000 – $10500 MXN	[$486 – $567 USD]
Botox:	$80 MXN per unit	[$4.32 USD]
Radio frequency facial (session):	$700 – $800 MXN	[$37.83 – $43.24 USD]

General practitioners

Consultation:	$150-$300 MXN	[$8.10 – $16.21 USD]

(There may be additional costs for certain procedures, medications and/or testing)

Gynecologist

Consultation:	$600 – $800 MXN	[$32.43 – $43.24 USD]
Pap Smear	$350 – $500 MXN	[$18.91 – $27.02 USD]

Lab work

In Mexico, you can go to a lab without a doctor's referral and receive a wide range of services. The following are only a few of the services they provide:

Pregnancy test:	$185 – $265 MXN	[$10 – $14.32 USD]

Prostate-specific antigen, or PSA:	$375 – $535 MXN	[$20.27 – $28.92 USD]
Glucose:	$85 – $120 MXN	[$4.59 – $6.49 USD]
Uric Acid:	$85 – $120 MXN	[$4.59 – $6.49 USD]
Cholesterol:	$115 – $165 MXN	[$6.22 – $8.92 USD]
Drug Testing:	$290 – $535 MXN	[$15.68 – $28.92 USD]
Standard blood tests:	$970 – $1510 MXN	[$52.43 – $81.62 USD]

Other Specialists

Cardiologist, pediatrician, orthopedist etc.

Consultation: $600 – $800 MXN   [$32.43 – $43.24 USD]

(There may be additional costs for certain procedures, medications and/or testing)

Pharmacies (Doctor on site)

Many pharmacies in Mexico have a *consultorio* with a medical doctor that handles minor injuries and illnesses. This is a fast, economical option if you are feeling a little under the weather while on vacation.

Consultation: $25-$50 MXN   [$1.35 – $2.70 USD]

(There may be additional costs for certain procedures, medications and/or testing)

X-Rays, ultrasounds, and MRI's

The price ranges are a little wider here because it depends on the complexity and type of the particular scan. For example, an ultrasound of your liver is $450 pesos but a ultrasound of the fetus in the womb is $940 pesos.

Ultrasounds :	$360 – $940 MXN	[$19.45 – $50.81 USD]
X-Rays:	$300 – $500 MXN	[$16.21 – $27.02 USD]
MRI:	$6000 – $8000 MXN	[$324.32 – $432.43 USD]

Appendix N: Alternative Medical Clinics in Mexico

Name: Angeles Functional Oncology
Approach: Integrative whole health
Treating: Cancer
Website: https://www.mexicancancerclinics.com/angeles-functional-oncology
Email: cancerclinicsmx@gmail.com
USA Phone: 619-751-8265
Mexico Address: Tijuana

Name: The Center for Holistic Life Extension
Approach: Autochemotherapy, live-cell therapy, nutrition, organ therapy, homeopathy, iridology, herb therapy
Treating: Cancer, immune system, degenerative illnesses, autoimmune disorders, allergies, asthma, substance abuse, collagen illness, bone & muscle system and more
Website: http://www.extendlife.com/
Email: http://www.extendlife.com/ask.php
USA Phone: 619-253-1995
Mexican Phone: 011 521 (664) 193-1997
USA Address: San Ysidro, CA

Name: Gerson Institute
Approach: Gerson Therapy, nutrition
Treating: Cancer, diabetes, heart disease, arthritis, auto-immune disorders, etc.
Website: https://gerson.org/gerpress/
Email: https://gerson.org/gerpress/email-form/
USA Phone: 619-685-5353
USA Address: San Diego
Mexico Address: Tijuana

Name: Heberprot-P: Centro de Atención al Pié Diabético
Approach: Heberprot-P
Treating: Diabetic foot ulcers
Website: www.heberprot-p.com.mx/
Facebook: https://www.facebook.com/Heberprot-P-Centro-de-Atención-al-Pié-Diabético-248501585173308/?fref=ts
Toll Free USA Phone: 01 844 439 0739
Mexico Address: Blvd. Venustiano Carranza # 4036 Torre 2 de especialidades, Consultorio Número 23, Saltillo, Mexico

Name: Hope4Cancer Institute
Approach: Virotherapy, detox, integrative, immunotherapy
Treating: Cancer
Website: http://www.hope4cancer.com/
Email: on site form
Toll Free USA Phone: 1-888-544-5993
USA/International Phone: +1-619-669-6511
USA Address: Jamul, CA (mailing address)
Mexico Address: Baja California, Mexico

Name: Hoxsey BioMedical Center
Approach: Hoxsey alternative to chemotherapy
Treating: Cancer
Website: http://www.hoxseybiomedical.com
Email: http://www.hoxseybiomedical.com/contact-us/
USA Phone: (619) 704 8442 – (619) 407 7858
Mexican Phone: 011 52 664 684 9011
Mexico Address: 3170 General Ferreira, Colonia Madero Sur, Tijuana, Baja California, Mexico

Name: Immunity Therapy Center
Approach: Oxygen Cancer Therapy, Insulin Potentiation Therapy (IPT), Rife Therapy,
Biomagnetic Cancer Therapy, IV Cancer Therapy, Regenerative Cell Cancer Therapy
Treating: Cancer, infectious diseases, autoimmune diseases, chronic degenerative diseases
Website: http://www.immunitytherapycenter.com/
Contact: http://www.immunitytherapycenter.com/contact/
USA Phone: 1-619-870-8002
Mexico Address: Tijuana, Mexico

Name: International BioCare Hospital & Wellness Center
Approach: Integrative, stem cell, hyperthermia
Treating: Cancer, Hepatitis C, chronic fatigue, autoimmune disease
Website: http://biocarehospital.com/
Email: doctor@biocarehospital.com.com
USA & Canada Phone: 800-701-7345
International Phone: 1-619-309-2080
Mexico Address: Tijuana

Name: Issels Immuno-Oncology
Approach: Integrative immunotherapy
Treating: Cancer
Website: http://issels.com/
Email: http://66.135.32.155/issels/Questionnaire/request-issels-info.aspx

Toll Free Phone: from USA and Canada 1-888-447-7357
Toll Free Phone: from abroad 001-888-447-7357
USA Address: Outpatient, Santa Barbara, California
Mexico Address: Inpatient, Tijuana

Name: Mexico HIFU
Approach: HIFU (High Intensity Focused Ultrasound)
Treating: Prostate cancer
Website: http://mexicohifu.com/
Email: info@hifumx.com
Mexico Phone: 52 (322) 2 21 27 77
Mexico Address: Timon 1-C , Marina Vallarta, Puerto Vallarta, México

Name: Oasis of Hope
Approach: Multi-disciplinary, laetrile/B17, AHCC, micronutrients, integrative, low-dose
chemotherapy, hyperthermia
Treating: Cancer
Website: http://www.oasisofhope.com/
Email: http://www.oasisofhope.com/
USA Phone: 1-619-690-8450
Toll Free Phone: 1-888-500-4673
Mexico Phone: +52 664 631 6100
Mexico Address: Paseo Playas de Tijuana 19 Fracc. Playas de Tijuana

Name: PanAm HIFU
Approach: HIFU (High Intensity Focused Ultrasound)
Treating: Prostate cancer
Website: http://www.panamhifu.com/
Email: http://www.panamhifu.com/contact.php
Toll Free USA Phone: 877-766-8400
USA Phone: 1-941-957-0007
USA Address: Sarasota, FL
Mexico Address: Cancun

Name: Pangea Biomedics
Approach: Ibogaine treatment
Treating: Opiate addiction
Website: http://pangeabiomedics.com
Email: info@pangeabiomedics.com
Skype: ibogaine1414
USA Phone: 801 405-6823
Mexico Address: Riviera Nayarit

Name: Regenerative Cellular Therapy (RCT)
Approach: Peptide and protein therapeutics
Treating: neurological diseases including Alzheimer's, brain injury, and dementia, and rheumatic conditions including arthritis and lupus
Website: http://www.rctherapy.net
Email: contact@rctherapy.net
USA Phone: 480-626-4845
Mexico Phone: 52 480-626-4845
Mexico Address: Puerto Penasco, Sonora, Mexico

Name: San Diego Clinic
Approach: Immunological therapies, integrative care
Treating: Cancer, chronic fatigue, diabetes, hypertension, metabolic syndrome, heart disease and more
Website: http://www.sdiegoclinic.com/
Email: http://www.sdiegoclinic.com/contact.html
USA Phone: +1.619-804-7783
Mexico Address: Tijuana

Name: Sanoviv Medical Institute
Approach: Integrative, holistic, detox, rigvir, nutrition
Treating: Cancer, chronic, degenerative and neurological conditions
Website: http://www.sanoviv.com/
Email: http://www.sanoviv.com/admission-form/firstContact/contact.html
Email: Inquiries@sanoviv.com
Toll Free USA Phone: 800-726-6848
Mexico Address: Baja California, Mexico

Name: St. Andrews Clinic
Approach: Antiangiogenic therapy, chelation, laetrile, hyperthermia, hydrogen peroxide IV, insulin potentiation
Treating: Cancer
Website: http://standrewsclinic.com/
Email: http://standrewsclinic.com/contact
USA Phone: 1-619-730-0787
Mexico Address: Tijuana

Name: Stella Maris Clinic
Approach: Metabolic therapies
Treating: Cancer
Website: http://stellamarisclinic.com/

Email: http://stellamarisclinic.com/contact_us.php
USA Phone: 619-405-5199
Mexican Phone: 011 52-664-634-3444
Mexico Address: Tijuana

Name: Dr. Ulises, surgeon
Approach: Heberprot-P
Treating: Diabetic foot ulcers
Website: https://www.blogger.com/profile/03721836599602261488
Wesbite: http://ulisesprieto.blogspot.mx/2010/11/heberprot-p-en-mexico-este-es-su-mes.html
Email: Ulises_prieto@hotmail.com
Mexico Phone: 52-971-128-1725 or 52-961-137-1092
Mexico Address: Juchitan de Zaragoza, Oaxaca, Mexico

Appendix O: Fertility Treatment Centers by State & City

Acapulco de Juárez

Acapulco de Juárez

Adan Oliveros Ceballos
La Nao No. 1809, Magallanes
01 74 44 88 11 14 y 0 / 01 74 44 87 68 38
cagyr@prodigy.net.mx
http://www.analisisdesemen.com.mx/

Baja California

León

Hospital Aranda de la Parra S.A de C.V.
Hidalgo No. 329, Centro
01(477)719-71-00 / 01(47)16-49-03
gerencia@arandadelaparra.com
http://www.arandadelaparra.com/2008/index.html

Instituto de Medicina Reproductiva del Bajio
Hidalgo 333-202, Centro
01(47)13-29-65/14-9

Instituto de Ciencias en Reproduccion Humana S.C.
Plaza Las Americas No. 115
01(477)779 08 35/3 / 01(477)779 08 35/3
http://www.institutovida.com/

Consultorio Medico de Especialidad en Reproducción Humana
Quetzales No. 141, San Isidro
01 477 7116206

Clinica Siena
Boulevard Campestre no. 306 1 Piso,
Consultorio 108, Jardines Del Moral

014777161910, 01477 / 014777161929
dr.francisco.hernandez@gmail.com
http://www.pronacer.com

Tijuana

Centro de Fertilidad del Noroeste, S.A. de C.V.
Bugambilias 50 No. 503, Del Prado
016846080262

OHA Sucursal Hospital Angeles Tijuana
Av. Paseo de los Heroes No. 10999, Zona Rio
01 664 635 19 00 ext / 01 664 635 19 15
crdgz@saludangeles.com

Chihuahua

Juárez

Clinica del Parque S.A. de C.V.
Pedro Leal Rodriquez No. 1802, Centro
01 614 439 79 79 / 01 614 439 79 20
clinicaparque@infosel.net.mx
http://www.hcp.com.mx

Distrito Federal (Mexico City)

Benito Juárez

OHA Sucursal Hospital Ángeles Metropolitano
Tlacotlalpan No. 59, Roma Sur
5265-1800 / 52 64 20 60
hector.baragan@saludangel

Instituto de Reproduccion Humana y Genetica
Pedro Rosales de León No. 7510, Fuentes del Valle
01 656 618 05 98 / 01 656 617 32 00
poliplaza@terra.com.mx
http://www.poliplaza.com/espanol/irhuge.html

Cuauhtémoc

Centro de Fertilidad Humana en Mexico S.A. de C.V.
Tuxpan No. 6-401 y 602, Roma Sur
5574-4677, 5574-918 / 5574-3018
cfhm@centrodefertilidad.com
http://www.centrodefertilidad.com

Laboratorio Fertimexico, S.A. de C.V.
Tuxpan No. 54-201, Roma Sur
http://www.analisisdesemen.com.mx/

Instituto de Infertilidad y Genética México, S.C.
Juan Salvador Agraz No. 40-3, Santa Fe
2789 9800
http://www.ingenes.com/

Gustavo. Madero
Hospital Médica Integra S.A. de C.V.
Managua #730, Lindavista
57 52 12 34

Magdalena Contreras, La

OHA Sucursal Hospital Ángeles Pedregal
Camino Santa Teresa No. 1055, Heroes de Padierna
5652-118 / 5652-8598 / 5449-550
ehuico@saludangeles.com

Proyectos Especiales A.G.N. S.A. de C.V.
Camino a Santa Teresa No. 1055-701,
7mo Piso, Heroes de Padierna
56-52-11-11/56-52-2 / 56-52-65-58
grygagn@terra.com.mx

Miguel Hidalgo

Reproduccion Asistida Metroplitana S.C.
Temistocles #210 Cuarto Piso, Chapultepec Morales
52 50 63 93 / 52 50 63 93
http://www.ram-mexico.com.mx/

Centro Especializado en Esterilidad y Reproducción Humana, S.C.

Agrarismo Núm 208, Torre"a" 1er. Piso
(Hospital Angeles de Mexico), Col. Escandon
5271 62 18 y 52 77-1 / 5271 62 18 y 52 77-1
http://www.ceerh.com.mx/index.htm

Laboratorio de Reproducción Asistida S.A. de C.V.
Av. De Las Palmas No. 745 Mezanine 3,
Lomas de Chapultepec
55206650 / 55202668
scuneo@concibe.com.mx
http://www.concibe.com.mx

Clinica Hisparep de Fertilidad Asistida
Av. Ejercito Nacional Mexicano No. 613-101, Granada
5250-6461 / 5250-646
http://www.hisparep.com.mx/index.html

Instituto Mexicano de Alta Tecnologia Reproductiva, S.C.
Bosque de Ciruelos No. 168 P.B.,
Bosques de las Lomas
52458169 / 52458194 ext. 102
imaldonado@inmater.com
http://www.inmater.com

Instituto Especializado en Infertilidad y Medicina Reproductiva (Insemer)
Avenida de las Palmas No. 735,
Piso 10, Consultorio No. 1001 y 1008,
Lomas de Chapultepec
http://insemer.com/

Tlalpan

Repromedica S.A. de C.V.
Puente de Piedra No. 150 Torre I C-514,
Toriello Guerra
56 66 81 76 / 56 66 81 76
http://www.analisisdesemen.com.mx/

Guanajuato

Celaya

Medica Fertil, S.A. de C.V. Morelia No. 405, Alameda
014616135010

Jalisco

Guadalajara

Unidad de Reproducción del Country, S.C.
Mar Marmara No. 1979,
Chapultepec Country
0133 38230145/54
unir_c@hotmail.com

Instituto Imer de Occidente, S.C. Pablo Neruda No. 3148,
Providencia Norma Patricia Ramos Gonzalez
Tarascos No. 3473-310, Rinconada Sta. Rita
Lab. 0133 3648 6266 / 0133 3642 6678
Pattram25@hotmail.com
http://www.institutoimer.com/html/main.htm

New Hope Fertility Center S. de RL de C.V.
Avenda Americas No. 1501-P 12 B,
Providencia
http://www.nhfc.mx/index.html
http://www.newhopefertility.com/dr-chavez-badiola-alejandro_dr-chavez-badiola.shtml

Zapopan

Instituto Mexicano de Infertilidad
Blvd Puerta de Hierro No. 5150 Int. 503-506,
Plaza Corporation Zapopan
013336482550 ext 1 ext 121 chanonafjc@hotmail.com
http://www.imimexico.com/

Instituto de Ciencias en Reproducción Humana de Guadalajara, S.C.
Av. Empresarios No. 150 PB, Puerta de Hierro
http://www.institutovida.com/Guadalajara.asp

Mexico

Centro

Centro de Cirugia Reproductiva y Ginecologia
Prolongación Usumacinta No. 2085-424, Tabasco 2000

Huixquilucan

Centro Especializado Para la Atención de la Mujer S.C.
Vialidad de la Barranca S/N,
Valle de las Palmas
01(55)52 46-94-10 / 01(55)52 46-94-11
info@cepam.com.mx

Naucalpan de Juárez

Cefam S. de R.L. de C.V.
Pafnuncio Padilla No. 43-8, Ciudad Satelite
http://www.cefam.com.mx/

Nuevo Leon

Monterrey

Clinica Ginecologia y Obstetricia S.A. de C.V.
(Monterrey) Av. Hidalgo No 1842 PTE., Obispado
01(81) 83 47 20 99 / 01(81) 83 47 20 40
iech@nl1/telmex.net.mx/rsa
http://www.iech.com.mx

Creasis, S.C.
Dr. Enrique Peña No. 118, Los Doctores
http://www.creasis.com.mx/index.shtml

Puebla

Puebla

Unidad de Reproduccion Humana

Privada 8 A Sur No. 2509, Ladrillera de Benitez
http://www.unidaddereproduccionhumana.com.mx/

Gyra de Puebla, S.C.
21 Poniente No. 3713,
Belisario Dominguez
http://www.gyra.com.mx/default.asp

Querétaro

Querétaro

Instituto Queretano de Fertilidad S.C.
Bernanrdino del Razo No. 21-215 C, Ensueño
(442)1923056
www.angeleshealth.com/

Medica Fertil, S.A. de C.V.
Prol. Constituyentes No. 218, El Jacal
014422154624
http://www.medicafertil.com.mx/pagina/uinfertilidad.html

Clinica Ginecologica y Medicina Reproductiva
Bernardo Quintana No. 305 Sur, Centro Sur
229 0154

San Luis Potosí

San Luis Potosi

Medica Fertil
Avenida Benito Juarez No. 4055,
Cuartel Casanova, Villa de Pozos
444 166 6809

Sinaloa

Culiacan

Centro Mexicano de Fertilidad

Blvd. Pedro Ma Anaya No. 2136-A,
Prol. Chapultepec, Culiacan
http://www.cemef.com.mx/

Sonora

Hermosillo

Hospital Privado de Hermosillo S.A. De C.V.
Paseo Rio San Miguel No. 35,
Proyecto Rio Sonora
01(6)259-09-00/59-0 / 01(6)259-09-99/59-0
jmojarra@rtn.uson.mx

Veracruz

Veracruz

Centro de Diagnóstico Ginecológico
Grijalba No. 174, Fracc. Reforma
01 229 937 6797 / 01 229 935 5629
oscar7enri@hotmail.com
http://cdgfertilidad.galeon.com/

Yucatán

Mérida

Instituto de Ciencias en Reproduccion Humana S.C.
Av. Colon No. 204-D, Garcia Gineres
01 999 925 30 20/925 / 01 999 925 30 20/925
vidamerida@hotmail.com
http://www.institutovida.com/

Appendix P: Accessible Travel Resources

Society for Accessible Travel and Hospitality - Dedicated to the needs of disabled travelers http://sath.org/

Accessible Journeys - Travel planning tips and arrangement of medical equipment rentals abroad http://www.disabilitytravel.com/accessible-travel-tips.htm

Mobility International USA - Resources for study, work, volunteer, teaching or cultural programs abroad http://www.miusa.org/

Wheelchair Accessible Travel Guide - Comprehensive information on how to plan travel with a wheelchair http://www.tripbuzz.com/wheelchair-accessible-travel-guide/

Persons with Disabilities Using Commercial Airlines for Travel - Resources for disabled travellers using commercial airlines http://www.defensetravel.dod.mil/site/faqdisable.cfm

Travelling Tips for People Living with Neuromuscular Disease - Checklist before you take off https://www.mda.org/sites/default/files/TravelingTips.pdf

Travel Tips for the Hearing Impaired - Preparation tips before you travel http://www.entnet.org/content/travel-tips-hearing-impaired

Canadian Transportation Agency - Guide for persons with disabilities - A comprehensive guide to help prepare you before you travel https://www.otc-cta.gc.ca/eng/take-charge

Disabled Travelers– Dedicated to providing a comprehensive listing of accessible travel specialists http://www.executiveclasstravelers.com/1/index.htm

Appendix Q: Placing Phone Calls To & Inside Mexico

Emergency calls in Mexico (National): 911
Hotel-placed long-distance calls can be very expensive. Ask the price before making the call.

Long Distance Calls to Mexico

- From within Mexico: 01 + city code + local number
- From the U.S. or Canada: 011 + 52 + city code + local number
- From other countries: international access code + 52 + city code + local number
- Calls to a cell phone from outside Mexico: omit the "044" which often prefixes a cell phone number

Long Distance Calls from Mexico

- To a Mexican telephone number: 01 + city code + local number
- To the U.S. or Canada: 001 + area code + local number
- To other countries: 00 + country code + city code + local number [191]
- To a cell phone in Mexico: 045 + area code + local number
- Operated-assisted calls in Mexico: 020
- Operated-assisted calls to other countries: 090

City Codes

Acapulco	744	La Paz	612	Santa Rosalia	615
Aguascalientes	449	Lagunas	972	Tecate	665
Campeche	981	Leon	477	Tijuana	664
Cancun	998	Manzanillo	314	Tlaxcala	246
Celaya	461	Mexicali	686	Todos Santos	612
Celestun	988	Mexico City	55	Toluca	722
Cihuatlan	315	Merida	999	Torreon	871
Ciudad Jimenez	629	Monterrey	81	Tulum	984
Ciudad Juarez	656	Morelia	443	Tuxtla Gutierrez	961
Colima	312	Oaxaca	951	Uruapan	452
Comitan	963	Pachuca	771	Valladolid	985
Cordoba	271	Puebla	222	Valparaiso	457
Cuernavaca	777	Puerto Vallarta	322	Veracruz	229
Culiacan	667	Salamanca	464	Villahermosa	993
Durango	618	Saltillo	844	Zacatecas	492
Guadalajara	33	San Cristobal	967	Zamora	351
Guanajuato	473	San Luis Potosi	444	Zitacuaro	715

Pay Phones

These typically use phone cards that are readily available in many small stores (for example, the OXXO chain of quick marts). They may be the least expensive way to call the United States or Canada.

044: Many cell phone numbers in Mexico have the prefix "044".

- This is only used when calling the number locally and is omitted for international calls. So, to place a call locally to a cell phone you must dial 044 + the 10-digit number.
- To place a long distance call to the cell phone you omit the 044, e.g. 011-52 + the 10-digit number.
- To place an international call to a cell phone, you now must add a "1" after the country code, i.e. 011-52-1 + 10-digit number.

Long Distance Within Mexico

If you are calling a Mexican cell phone from within Mexico but it is a long distance call—

- Dial the prefix is 045; then dial the 10-digit number.
- Omit the 045 when calling from outside Mexico and dial 011-52 + the 10-digit number.

Endnote

1 http://relentlesslycreativebooks.com/?mbt_book=the-english-speakers-guide-to-doctors-hospitals-in-mexico

2 http://primeroslibros.org/page_view.php?id=pl_bjml_004&lang=es&page=1

3 http://economix.blogs.nytimes.com/2009/07/15/how-much-do-doctors-in-other-countries-make/?_r=0

4 http://www.worldsalaries.org/mexico.shtml

5 https://dl.dropboxusercontent.com/u/21505415/travel_history_form.pdf

6 http://www.seguro-popular.salud.gob.mx/images/Contenidos/gestion/ANEXO%20I%202016.pdf

7 https://www.apostille.us/Documents/Document_Birth_Certificate.shtml

8 http://www.seguro-popular.salud.gob.mx/index.php?option=com_content&view=article&id=100&Itemid=137

9 http://www.sandiegoleisure.com/files/CURP2.pdf

10 https://consultas.curp.gob.mx/CurpSP/

11 http://www.cedulaprofesional.sep.gob.mx/cedula/presidencia/indexAvanzada.action

12 https://mx.usembassy.gov/embassy-consulates/embassy/

13 http://www.canadainternational.gc.ca/mexico-mexique/index.aspx?lang=eng

14 https://www.gov.uk/government/world/mexico

15
https://play.google.com/store/apps/details?id=com.dgis.radarcisaludhttps://play.google.com/store/apps/details?id=com.dgis.radarcisalud

16 https://itunes.apple.com/mx/app/radarcisalud/id1057984642?mt=8

17 http://www.rxlist.com/script/main/hp.asp

18 http://www.anadim.com.mx/index.php

19 http://www.peoplesguide.com/1pages/chapts/health/buymed/cheapmeds2.html

20 http://relentlesslycreativebooks.com/?mbt_book=the-english-speakers-guide-to-doctors-hospitals-in-mexico

21 http://relentlesslycreativebooks.com/?mbt_book=the-english-speakers-guide-to-doctors-hospitals-in-mexico

22 https://www.ethno-botanik.org/Heilpflanzen/Medicinal-plants-Mexico.html

23 http://www.seguros-insurance.net/

24 https://apps.allianzworldwidecare.com/poi/hospital-doctor-and-health-practitioner-finder?COUNTRY=Mexico&amp%3bCON=Central_America

25 http://www.seguros-insurance.net/

26 http://www.rand.org/pubs/occasional_papers/OP314.html

[27] https://medicavrim.com/index.aspx

[28] http://www.medicallhome.com/MedicallHomeWeb/

[29] info@doctorsandhospitalsinmexico.com

[30] http://www.diputados.gob.mx/LeyesBiblio/ref/lgs/LGS_ref39_05ene09.pdf

[31] https://www.hrw.org/news/2014/10/24/mexico-needless-suffering-end-life

[32] http://rollybrook.com/life_care_law.htm

[33] http://www.diputados.gob.mx/LeyesBiblio/ref/lgs/LGS_ref39_05ene09.pdf

[34] http://hospicecare.com/global-directory-of-providers-organizations/

[35] http://www.medtogo.com/

[36] http://cabohealthtravel.com/

[37] http://www.gob.mx/cenatra

[38] http://bit.ly/163JS3Q

[39] http://www.cancerdecisions.com/

[40] https://issuu.com/drkandrew/docs/tijuana-cancer-clinics-in-the-post-nafta-era

[41] http://www.acc.org/latest-in-cardiology/articles/2016/02/26/09/34/chelation-therapy-for-cad?w_nav=TI

[42] http://www.huffingtonpost.com/gail-reed/renewed-uscuba-relations-_b_6537518.html

[43] http://abcnews.go.com/Health/story?id=4537744&page=1

[44] https://www.drugabuse.gov/about-nida/legislative-activities/testimony-to-congress/2015/americas-addiction-to-opioids-heroin-prescription-drug-abuse

[45] http://www.theverge.com/2015/11/11/9700446/ibogaine-treatment-opiate-addiction-psychedelic-drug

[46] http://www.thedailynewsonline.com/bdn01/going-abroad-for-the-cure-man-with-ms-seeks-procedure-in-mexico-20160617

[47] https://draxe.com/vitamin-b17/

[48] http://laligadelaleche.org.mx/

[49] https://www.plannedparenthood.org/learn/morning-after-pill-emergency-contraception

[50] http://www.npr.org/sections/health-shots/2016/06/09/481269789/legal-medical-abortions-are-up-in-texas-but-so-are-diy-pills-from-mexico

[51] https://safe2choose.org/abortion-pill/using-mifepristone-and-misoprostol/

[52] http://www.nydailynews.com/news/national/arizona-woman-feeling-pain-83-046-bill-anti-venom-drug-seeking-medical-treatment-scorpion-sting-article-1.1152754

[53] https://www.iamat.org/

[54] http://www.istm.org/

[55] https://www.verywell.com/ibd-crohns-colitis-treatment-4014257

56 http://sls.org/project/directory-of-sls-members/

57 https://www.iamat.org/elibrary/view/id/1388

58 https://www.iamat.org/elibrary/view/id/1359

59 https://www.iamat.org/elibrary/view/id/1378

60 http://www.paho.org/hq/index.php?option=com_topics&view=article&id=343&Itemid=40931&lang=en

61 https://www.iamat.org/risks/zika-virus

62 https://www.iamat.org/risks/dengue

63 https://www.iamat.org/insect-bite-prevention

64 http://www.paho.org/hq/index.php?option=com_topics&view=article&id=1&Itemid=40734

65 https://www.iamat.org/risks/zika-virus

66 https://www.iamat.org/risks/yellow-fever

67 https://www.iamat.org/risks/west-nile-virus

68 https://www.iamat.org/risks/japanese-encephalitis

69 https://www.iamat.org/risks/chikungunya

70 https://www.iamat.org/risks/zika-virus

71 https://www.iamat.org/risks/yellow-fever

72 https://www.iamat.org/insect-bite-prevention

73 http://www.iamat.org/elibrary/view/id/2968

74 http://www.iamat.org/elibrary/view/id/1376

75 https://www.iamat.org/assets/files/How%20to%20Protect%20Yourself%20Against%20Malaria%202015b.pdf

76 https://www.iamat.org/risks/zika-virus

77 https://www.iamat.org/risks/hepatitis-b

78 http://www.hivtravel.org/

79 https://www.iamat.org/elibrary/view/id/1391

80 https://www.iamat.org/elibrary/view/id/1392

81 https://www.iamat.org/elibrary/view/id/1398

82 http://www.paho.org/hq/index.php?option=com_content&view=article&id=11585&Itemid=41688&lang=en

83 https://www.iamat.org/risks/dengue

84 https://www.iamat.org/risks/yellow-fever

85 https://www.iamat.org/risks/west-nile-virus

86 https://www.iamat.org/risks/japanese-encephalitis

[87] https://www.iamat.org/risks/dengue

[88] https://www.iamat.org/risks/chikungunya

[89] http://www.iamat.org/pdf/Mental_Health_TravelStress.pdf

[90] http://www.iamat.org/pdf/Mental_Health_Depression.pdf

[91] http://www.iamat.org/pdf/Mental_Health_Anxiety.pdf

[92] http://www.iamat.org/pdf/Mental_Health_Psychosis.pdf

[93] https://www.iamat.org/

[94] http://www.rocketlanguages.com/spanish/premium/?aff=clickixax&type=freetrial

[95] http://www.aamexico.org.mx/

[96] http://www.na.org/MeetingSearch/

[97] http://www.gob.mx/profeco

[98] http://www.gob.mx/conamed

[99] http://www.cedulaprofesional.sep.gob.mx/cedula/presidencia/indexAvanzada.action

[100] http://relentlesslycreativevbooks.com

[101] http://www.mexperience.com/store/vuitem.php?itemid=41

[102] http://relentlesslycreativebooks.com/?mbt_book=the-english-speakers-guide-to-doctors-hospitals-in-mexico

[103] http://www.compedia.org.mx/

[104] http://cmica.org.mx/

[105] http://www.cma.org.mx/

[106] http://www.cmacv.org.mx/

[107] http://amcaofmexico.org/

[108] http://www.smcardiologia.org.mx/

[109] https://ancam.org.mx/

[110] http://coloproctologia-mexico.org/

[111] http://www.amcpc.org.mx/

[112] http://cmmcritica.org.mx/

[113] http://www.amd.org.mx/

[114] http://www.consejomexicanodermatologia.org.mx/

[115] http://www.amd.org.mx/

[116] http://www.cmmu.org.mx/

[117] https://www.endocrinologia.org.mx/

[118] http://www.facmed.unam.mx/deptos/familiar/

[119] http://www.colegiomexicanodemedicinafamiliar.org/

[120] http://cmgastro.org.mx/

[121] https://www.gastro.org.mx/

[122] http://www.cmgac.org.mx/

[123] http://consejomexicanodegeriatria.org/

[124] http://www.femecog.org.mx/

[125] http://www.cmgo.org.mx/cmgo/

[126] http://www.cmhematologia.org/

[127] http://www.amimc.org.mx /

[128] http://sminmunologia.org/

[129] http://www.compedia.org.mx/

[130] http://www.cmmi.org.mx/

[131] http://www.consejomexicanodenefrologia.org/

[132] http://www.neurologia.org.mx/

[133] http://www.consejomexicanodeneurologia.org/

[134] http://www.cmnfc.org/

[135] http://cmmn.org.mx/

[136] http://www.cnmmt.mx/

[137] http://www.smeo.org.mx /

[138] http://www.cmo.org.mx/

[139] http://www.smo.org.mx/

[140] http://cmoftalmologia.org/

[141] http://www.cmorlccc.org.mx/

[142] http://www.compac.org.mx/

[143] http://www.consejomexicanodemedicosanatomopatologos.org/

[144] http://www.cmcpmx.org/

[145] http://www.compedia.org.mx/

[146] http://www.consejorehabilitacion.org.mx/index.php

[147] http://www.consejonacionaldeneumologia.org.mx/

[148] http://consejomexicanopsiquiatria.org.mx/

[149] http://www.sociedadmexicanadepsicologia.org/

[150] http://www.smsp.org.mx/

[151] http://www.fmri.org.mx/

[152] http://www.cmri.org.mx/

[153] http://www.consejoreumatologia.org/

[154] http://www.conamede.org.mx/web/

[155] http://www.smcrc.org.mx/

[156] http://www.consejo-cmeecr.com.mx/

[157] http://cnct.com.mx/

[158] http://amcg.org.mx/

[159] http://cmcgac.org.mx/

[160] http://karolldesig5.wixsite.com/comf

[161] http://www.smxcn.org/

[162] http://smo.edu.mx/

[163] http://femecot.org.mx/

[164] https://socmexcirped.org/

[165] http://www.cmcp.org.mx/

[166] http://cirugiaplastica.mx/

[167] http://www.cmcper.org.mx/

[168] http://www.conameu.org.mx/

[169] http://www.buap.mx/

[170] http://www.xochicalco.edu.mx/

[171] http://www.cicsma.ipn.mx/

[172] http://www.enmh.ipn.mx/

[173] http://www.esm.ipn.mx/

[174] http://www.itesm.mx/wps/wcm/connect/Campus/MTY/Monterrey/

[175] http://www.anahuac.mx/

[176] http://www.uabjo.mx/

[177] http://www.uaa.mx/

[178] http://www.facmed.unam.mx/

[179] http://www.facmed.unam.mx/

[180] http://uacam.mx/

[181] http://www.facmed.unach.mx/

[182] http://uach.mx/

[183] http://www.uacj.mx/

[184] http://www.uadec.mx/

[185] http://www.uadec.mx/

[186] http://www.uag.edu/

[187] http://www.uan.edu.mx/

[188] http://www.medicina.uanl.mx/

[189] http://www.uaq.mx/medicina/

[190] http://qroo.us/2016/07/08/mexico-a-look-at-the-costs-of-medical-and-dental-treatment/

[191] http://dialcodesplus.com/

Index

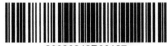

30090843R00137

Made in the USA
San Bernardino, CA
21 March 2019